Essential Oils & Weight Loss, Apple Cider Vinegar, Body Butters, Homemade Body Scrubs & Masks for Beginners & Coconut Oil for Easy Weight Loss

BY LINDSEY P

Book 1:

Essential Oils & Weight Loss for Beginners

&

Book 2:

Apple Cider Vinegar for Beginners

&

Book 3:

Body Butters for Beginners

&

Book 4:

Coconut Oil For Easy Weight Loss

&

Book 5:

Homemade Body Scrubs & Masks for Beginners

Book 1:

Essential Oils & Weight Loss for Beginners

BY LINDSEY P

Ultimate Guide to Losing Weight, Increasing Energy, Balancing Metabolism & Appetite Using Essential Oils & Aromatherapy

Essential Oils
&
Weight Loss
For Beginners

Ultimate Guide to Losing Weight, Increasing
Energy, Balancing Metabolism & Appetite Using
Essential Oils and Aromatherapy

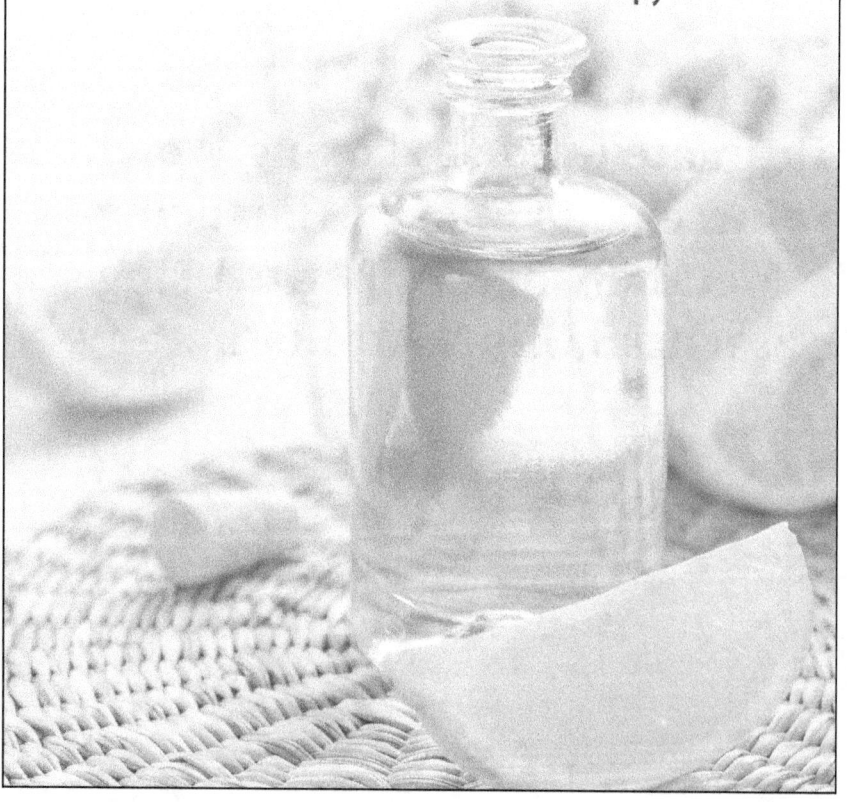

Table Of Contents

Introduction

I want to thank you and congratulate you for purchasing the book, "Essential Oils & Weight Loss for Beginners".

This book contains proven steps and strategies on how to make essentials oils work for you to help you conquer the battle against the weighing scale and measuring tape and to increase your energy and balance your metabolism.

It might sound a little far-fetched to hear that certain essential oils can actually help you to fight off your bulges. However, it is indeed possible! By the end of reading this book, you will find yourself more prepared and equipped to make essential oils work to your advantage. Read on to find out how orange peel essential oils can help turn your orange-peel skin into a cellulite-free smooth and toned skin.

Thanks again for purchasing this book, I hope you enjoy it!

Chapter 1: Essential Oils Basics

Before you get to learn which essential oils can help you in weight loss and how these can accomplish that, let us discuss first just what exactly essential oils are.

Essential oils are concentrated liquids that have a tendency to not absorb water or to not dissolve in or mix with water, it also has botanical aroma compounds that evaporate readily at normal temperature or pressure.

Oils from different kinds of plants are termed "essential" because it contains the essence or specific scent of the plant from which it was taken. It does not mean that it is essential or a must for one's health, but it sure can help us in more ways than one.

Distillation is the most common way used to extract essential oils from plants. Lavender, peppermint, and eucalyptus essential oils are the most commonly distilled oils. The different parts of the plant where the extract is to be taken from, like the roots, leaves, flowers, and others, are put inside a distillation apparatus, known as an alembic. It is then put over water and then heated. As the water's temperature rises, it will produce steam that will pass through the part of the plant, which will then vaporize the volatile elements in it. Then the vaporized compounds will then flow through a cooling coil, which will make it condense and return to a liquid state. Then the extracted liquid will then be collected in a container.

The less common processes are expression, which involves pressing the plants in a pressing device or machine to squeeze out the oils. Most citrus peels, like orange, lemon, and grapefruit, are expressed to get their essential oils. They can either be pressed mechanically or through cold-press. The peel of citrus fruits yield a large quantity of oil. In addition, growing and harvesting them takes very low cost. For this reason, essential oils from citrus fruits are less expensive compared to the cost of other essential oils.

Another way to get essential oils from plants is solvent extraction, which involves separating compounds using a funnel that separates it into two different liquids depending on their solubility. Most commonly, flowers undergo this process as they do not have enough volatile compounds for expression. Moreover, the chemical elements of flowers are too delicate and are readily denatured when heated at high temperatures using the process of steam distillation. Therefore, extraction through the use of solvents such as supercritical carbon dioxide is used to get the oils from the flowers.

Essential oils, also known as plant extracts, are used in cosmetics, soaps, perfumes, food and beverage flavoring, and other scented products. Although essential oils are not a requirement for the health, these have been applied medically throughout history as hair and skin treatments, cancer cures, aromatherapy, and others.

Western and Oriental medicine practitioners often argue about the efficacy of essential oils. Oriental or alternative medicine claims essential oils as having curative effects and many can testify to having been directly benefited by essential oils. When giving or being given acupressure or different kinds of massages, essential oils are used directly on the skin to be absorbed through the pores or diffused by nebulizers or burned as a candle or incense to be absorbed through the lungs.

If you would like to know how certain essential oils can help you to increase your metabolism, boost your energy, and help you lose weight, then please read on to the next chapter.

Chapter 2: How They Work for You

It is absolutely true that using certain essential oils can help you burn fat. However, nothing quite beats good old-fashioned proper diet and exercise. Discretion should be used when using essential oils to aid in weight loss. Never should one imagine or expect that certain essential oils are enough to keep your body fit and trimmed while you overeat and under-exercise.

That being said though, essential oils coupled with proper diet and exercise can do wonders for your body. Losing weight is not just about what you eat or what you do. It is also about how you feel about your body and about yourself.

Certain essential oils can help you when you are overeating because of certain events or experiences in your life. Let's face it. We eat our feelings every now and then. Whenever we are sorely distressed over something, we will almost instantly head to our favorite comfort food restaurant or food stall to eat a devilishly delicious and decadent chocolate cake or some hot and crispy deep fried poultry and root crops. Whichever the case, essential oils can give you comfort from whatever it is you are going through that makes you overeat with zero calories.

There are no particular essential oils that burn fat directly. However, certain essential oils can boost your metabolism, which in turn can help you in your weight loss goal and in cutting your body's fat deposits. Therefore, you must choose essential oils that aid in boosting your energy and metabolism.

Some of these energy-boosting and metabolism-balancing essential oils include citrus fruits (like oranges, lemons, bergamot, and grapefruits), herbs (like rosemary, sandalwood, and basil), and spices (like ginger, peppermint, and cinnamon).

There are many different ways in which you can mix and use these essential oils to your benefit depending on what you need them for. In the next chapter, we will talk about essential oils from citrus fruits.

Chapter 3: Citrus Essential Oils

It has long been proven by scientists that there is a strong link between what you smell, how you feel, and what eating pattern you have. Often, we take our senses for granted and do not realize just how strongly it affects our brain and behavior. You would agree that there is more than one time when your stomach grumbles like it is hungry when in fact, you just ate a short while ago and you are not actually hungry. Steadily inhaling citrus scents can help deceive our brain into thinking that our stomachs are full and therefore stopping it from sending signals to the brain that it is hungry.

The citrus family is a huge family. Citrus fruits have always benefited mankind in more ways than one. In this chapter, we will highlight the weight loss benefits of using essential oils from citrus fruits.

ORANGE. First on our list is the humble yet mighty and versatile orange. Different types of orange peels can yield their essential oils through the process of cold expression. Essential oils from different kinds of oranges are the most commonly added ingredients to various beauty products. Anti-aging creams, energizing body lotions, refreshing body wash variants, and other body care products use orange essential oils. Likewise, household items such as scented candles, aerosol deodorizing sprays for the rooms, and other scented products use orange essential oils.

Orange essential oils are also quite often used in pastries and other types of dishes as a flavoring and you would have ingested it more often than you are aware of. That being said though, you might become skeptical as to the efficacy of it since you have not felt directly any of its supposed properties in aiding you to lose weight and control your appetite.

The main reason for this is that the amount you absorb or consume is not enough for you to be able to feel the supposed effects. It can only act as a mood booster but that is pretty much the best you can get out of it. In order for you to feel the weight loss benefits, the orange essential oil must be in pure organic and undiluted form. That is why it is important to buy the pure, undiluted oils from trusted organic sources.

However, you must not confuse the fruit with the oil. The orange fruit is absolutely delicious and refreshing to the taste buds to eat. But the pure, undiluted orange oil is not to be eaten the way you would the fruit. To be able to benefit from the oil, you must use it in an aromatherapy session to help you control your cravings and cope with the everyday stress you encounter that might lead you to overeat.

You can put the orange essential oil in a diffuser to give a lingering, pleasant scent that everyone in the room can savor while the scent fills the room. If you are out and about, you can also bring a portable diffuser or inhaler so you can steadily inhale the refreshing scent of oranges for about five minutes to curb your cravings anytime you get them.

GRAPEFRUIT. The next one in line in the citrus family is the grapefruit. Grapefruit essential oils can stop your body from retaining water, which is one of the main causes of bloating, and can also dissolve fat in the body. The essential oil accomplishes this by releasing the stored fat into the bloodstream so your body can dissolve and absorb it and turn it into energy, helping you to feel energized. So you can say goodbye to your cellulites and say hello to toned thighs and arms.

Like orange essential oils, grapefruit essential oils can also be a strong suppressant for your cravings. It can help you feel fuller for longer. You can put a few drops of the grapefruit essential oil into your diffuser or inhaler to stop any hunger pangs from making you reach for another bag of chips. Another way is to put a drop of the essential oil in 8 ounces of drinking water to drink before you have your lunch or dinner. This will stop you from eating more than you should.

Grapefruit essential oils also help uplift your thoughts and moods. Improved moods can help you deal with stress better and help you have a better acceptance of yourself and your body, which can save you from developing any eating disorders, be it eating too much or too little.

You can mix different essentials oils as well to achieve better results. When you encounter extra stressful days that make you want to dive into a tub of vanilla ice cream, why not dive into your bath tub instead? Try mixing about eight drops of grapefruit essential oil and five drops of ginger essential oil to about two ounces of olive or sweet almond oil into your bath water and soak away to refreshment and relaxation.

The different essential oils you can mix together to relieve stress are lemon, chamomile, lavender, grapefruit, and jasmine essential oils. These essential oils have a calming effect. If you are depressed, uplifting and mood-boosting mixes can be of rose, sandalwood, orange, lavender, grapefruit, and jasmine essential oils. If you are feeling anxious, you can arrange for a massage and add a mixture or bergamot, sandalwood, rose, and lavender to your massage oil or as an incense to chase your anxieties away.

LEMON. Lemon essential oil is extracted from lemon rinds using cold press. It gently detoxifies the body. It relieves the body of some intestinal parasites that contribute to ill digestive health. Lemon has the ability to cleanse the body from toxins because of the antioxidant limonene. You can add a drop of lemon essential oil in a glass of water for a refreshing and uplifting drink. As with the abovementioned citrus fruits, lemon essential oil shares the same benefits for people wanting to lose weight and control their eating habits.

BERGAMOT. Bergamot is about the size of a typical orange but with a yellow rind like a lemon's. It is also used in many medicinal concoctions. Bergamot essential oils are strongly sedative and is therefore calming and best to use when you are stressed or tense that you want to reach for something decadent. So instead of letting sweets and simple sugars calm your nerves, let bergamot essential oils work for you. You will get the same calming effect without any added calories to your diet.

When paired with lavender essential oils, the calming or sedative effect will be more powerful. You can take a clean cloth and put a few drops of bergamot on it then steadily inhale it to help you relax when you are stressed out or when you get the urge to eat when you know you shouldn't. You can also dilute a drop of the oil in a teaspoon of honey and take it as you would cough syrup. Or you can make a calming yet delicious drink by diluting a drop of the oil in a small glass of almond or soy milk.

Well, now that you are acquainted with the citrus family, let us now get to know the other essential oils that will become your best friends in your war against cellulites.

Chapter 4: Non-citrus Essential Oils

In this chapter, we are going to talk about the not-so-citrus essential oils and how they can help us in expelling adipose tissues that are overstaying in our bodies.

PEPPERMINT. There is a part of your brain that tells you that your stomach is now filled with your mother's special meatloaf and that it can't accommodate anymore meatloaf. But sometimes, or should I say most of the time, we ignore what our brain tells us and listen to our eyes and taste buds telling us to eat more. Peppermint specifically works on that part of your brain to make it keep telling you that you are indeed full.

In addition, your tummy will love peppermint because it has proven itself as a great helper for digestion. It resolves a wide variety of digestive ailments. It can help you out if you are having problems with candida, as it is often a big influence in your losing or gaining weight. Moreover, when you are under heavy emotions like depression or anxiety, it can uplift and lighten your mood and motivate you to be more optimistic. And most importantly, peppermint tastes amazing and will let you give a minty fresh kiss to your special someone as well.

Before you eat anything, put a couple of drops of peppermint essential oil to a clean cloth or a cotton pad and steadily breathe in vapors. You can also put the drops in a diffuser and inhale your way to a reduced appetite. Likewise, you can put a drop of the peppermint oil in a glass of water for a refreshing drink before each meal. You can also pair it with lemon to get the most energizing and waistline-reducing effect.

SANDALWOOD. Sandalwood essential oils also have calming sedative properties that can help you control your eating habits when you are undergoing stressful situations. Sandalwood helps you combat negative feelings and actions. The feeling of having conquered negativity with relieve you of the stress you were having and so relieving you as well of the impulse to eat something comforting like you beloved mother's macaroni and cheese.

Sandalwood essential oils may be used with a diffuser and constantly inhaling the vapors. You can also dilute a drop of the sandalwood oil in a drop of extra virgin olive oil and then apply it directly on your feet or stomach for faster absorption. You can also take it like you would any medical syrup by adding a drop of sandalwood essential oil to a teaspoon of honey. You can also make a delicious drink by mixing a drop of the sandalwood oil to a small glass of rice milk.

GINGER. The lowly ginger is quite famous in Asian cuisine for being tummy-friendly. It is this spicy yet mildly sweet ingredient that makes Asian dishes taste really good. But its being tummy-friendly is not just because it makes dishes taste awesome. It is also loved by your stomach because of its anti-inflammatory and anti-bacterial properties that makes the stomach healthy and in tip-top shape.

In addition, ginger also has a warming effect on the body because of its being mildly spicy, stimulating the body, especially the nervous system. Ginger essential oil has been dubbed as the "oil of empowerment" as it gives off a mild heat that stimulates our inner strength, energizing and empowering the body and the mind.

To get the full benefit of ginger essential oil, you can put a couple of drops in a diffuser and inhale the vapors as you would any other essential oils that we have already discussed. You can also apply it directly to your skin or by diluting it first in coconut oil if you have sensitive skin. You can do a skin test first by applying it to your forearm to see if you are sensitive to it or not.

CINNAMON. Cinnamon is known to increase the weight loss effectiveness of all the other essential oils you have read about in this book. Diabetics can find comfort in knowing that cinnamon has been discovered to trigger healthy levels of insulin in the body. It also improves digestion and blood circulation. Its antioxidant properties help in gently detoxifying the body and stimulating the immune system to get to fight against invaders that try to give us colds and flu.

Cinnamon essential oil taken from the cinnamon leaves and twigs through steam distillation has a mildly spicy and musky scent. Cinnamon is great in aromatherapy. However, cinnamon oil from the cinnamon bark in not usually used in aromatherapy. Much like ginger essential oils, cinnamon essential oils are also mildly spicy and so it warms up the body as well and fights against exhaustion and depression by empowering the body.

In aromatherapy, you can put a few drops of the cinnamon essential oil in burners or vaporizers to be inhaled steadily to calm you and take your mind off eating out of stress. You can also dilute the oil in your bath water as you soak all your worries away. In addition, you can also simultaneously fight off any outwardly infections while soaking in your cinnamon infused bath water because of the cinnamon oil's antiseptic properties.

Chapter 5: A Helper and Complement

These essential oils that we have discussed in this book will only be effective if you work hard at your goal as well. Remember that nothing can replace proper diet and regular exercise to help you keep fit and healthy. But these essential oils can greatly help you in your struggle against whether to pick up that mouth-watering sandwich and take a bite off of it when you are not genuinely hungry.

These previously mentioned essential oils will boost you the two other main weapons in your war against excess fat. These essential oils have different properties that work to help you in breaking down fat in order to be fully absorbed by your body and turned into energy. They help curb your appetite and your "midnight-snack" cravings. They affect the part of the brain to help you relax and calm down instead of converting your anxieties and stresses into overeating.

Of course, disciplining yourself to eat the right kinds of food and to have a regular exercise program is difficult at first. You might be dreading or avoiding having to eat healthy food or having to go to the gym or just increase your daily physical activity. It might be the very reason that you have bought this book trying to find a way to lose weight without having to follow a proper diet and a regular exercise plan.

Well, following the instructions above and using essential oils alone in your goal of losing weight is indeed a possibility. It is not impossible. However, it is not enough and all the more so if you continue to live a sedentary lifestyle and choose unhealthy kinds of food. There should be balance in everything. One way or another, you are going to have to face the consequences of your actions (or for that matter, lack of action).

It is not at all daunting to follow a proper diet plan and a regular exercise program. But first, you have to want to make yourself healthier. Without your will and motivation, you most probably will not succeed. Moreover, you need to be consistent and steady with your routine to reach your goal of losing weight and keeping fit. If you are not consistent, you will undergo a yo-yo pattern, in which you will lose weight when you are motivated and gain weight when you are not.

It is not only bad for your health, it is also bad for your physical appearance as well because a yo-yo diet will ruin the elasticity of your skin causing it to have stretch marks and that will not be a very nice sight to see. Losing weight gradually coupled with good exercise will give your skin time to adjust to fit your new size, reducing the possibility of stretch marks and skin flaps that are commonly seen in people undergoing crash diets.

The food you eat also plays a big role in your goal to losing weight. Aside from keeping your body healthy in general, vitamins in fruits and vegetables, particularly vitamins A and E, will greatly increase your skins elasticity and give you a rosy glow on your cheeks suggesting you are indeed in the "pink of health".

The essential oils discussed in this book will be your ally in keeping a regular exercise routine. Orange and peppermint essential oils will perk you up and keep you feeling energized and motivated to follow your exercise program. Cinnamon and ginger essential oils will empower you to keep going even when you feel like you can't go on anymore.

Sandalwood and bergamot essential oils will calm and relax your nerves when you are feeling stressed out so you can win against the temptations of rich desserts and deep fried foods. And the best part about these essential oils is that it gives no side effects as it is pure and having no caffeine, no sugar, no preservatives.

A word of caution though. You may find some shops selling essential oils, usually containing a mixture of grapefruit, coconut, cedar, and other essential oils, claiming to burn fat. It would be great for calming and energizing you as discussed above. However, these cannot really help you to break down fat or cellulite in your body. It may temporarily make your skin look firmer because it hydrates your skin, but it is not a permanent fix.

It is better to research and experiment about which aromatherapy works best for you. Make sure that you do your homework and that you know how to properly use diffusers or inhalers to get the best out of your essential oils. When applying the essential oils directly on your body, make sure you dilute it first in a carrier oil such as virgin olive oil or coconut oil. Remember as well that some essential oils can be toxic to you if you directly ingest it. Always keep them in a safe place away from young children. Unless you have been using the essential oils for some time, only follow specific recipes to make sure it is safe for you.

Chapter 6: A Look in the Mirror

A mirror helps you to see yourself to check if you need to adjust your tie, if you need to reapply your lipstick, or if you have a piece of red bell pepper stuck to your teeth. But sometimes people forget to look at their inner mirror to check if the way they think or see things is correct. You need to take a good long look at yourself as well.

You need to honestly ask yourself whether you are doing this for yourself, to make yourself a better and healthier person or whether you are doing this just to please someone else. It is true that you need to present yourself well and make sure you look presentable when dealing with other people. But you should not change yourself just to please someone who does not genuinely care about you.

The motivation to lose weight should come from you, not from somebody else. Moreover, you should do it for the right reasons. When you are guided by a proper motivation and you have the right reasons to embark on the journey to weight loss, you will have more stability and consistency all throughout.

You will have a reason to go on even when you encounter setbacks in your goals, such as an unexpected dinner celebration for your friend's promotion or a relapse into pigging out during a family reunion, which ruins your carefully planned out diet, or a surprise added workload, which meant you would have to give up going to the gym for a few days to accommodate the added workload.

You need to be able to motivate yourself to continue even when setbacks happen. However, you will not always be strong.

Therefore, having a loved one or a friend know of your goals and asking for their support will greatly help you win the war against your bulges. You can also have a "weight loss buddy" whom you can be with as you journey towards a better health and a better self.

Having someone to exercise and eat proper amounts and right kinds of food with will make exercising and dieting less boring and tiresome. Knowing that you are in this together will empower you more while you let the essential oils work their magic to boost your energy. You can take essential oil-infused baths together or have your massages using your favorite essential oils together.

Not only will you be benefited by your regular exercise program, your proper healthy diet, and the essential oils we have discussed in this book, but you will also be benefited by the soothing and calming effect of human connection. All these things add up to make your whole weight loss journey more pleasant. Remember that those are puzzle pieces that need to be put together in order for you to complete the picture.

Conclusion

Thank you again for purchasing this book!

I hope this book was able to help you to realize the hidden potential of certain essential oils in weight loss, in increasing your body's energy, in uplifting your mood and countenance, and in improving your overall well-being.

The next step is to apply what you have learned in this book and to get you going on your way to physical fitness and better health. Remember that these facts about the essential oils mentioned above will be useless if you do not work hard and work steady. Avoid the yo-yo and crash diets. Slow and steady wins the race too. And in the race to weight loss, the fast and furious method won't really cut it. Take your time and enjoy your journey to a thinner and more healthy you!

Finally, if you enjoyed this book, please take the time to share your thoughts and post a review on Amazon. We do our best to reach out to readers and provide the best value we can. Your positive review will help us achieve that. It'd be greatly appreciated!

Thank you and good luck!

Book 2:
Apple Cider Vinegar for Beginners

BY LINDSEY P

Proven Secrets Using Apple Cider Vinegar for Health, Weight Loss, and Skin Care

APPLE CIDER VINEGAR FOR BEGINNERS

Proven Secrets using Apple Cider Vinegar for Health, Weight Loss, Skin and Hair Care

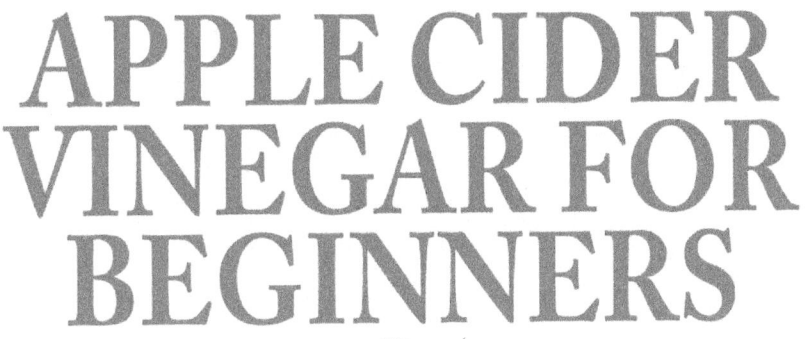

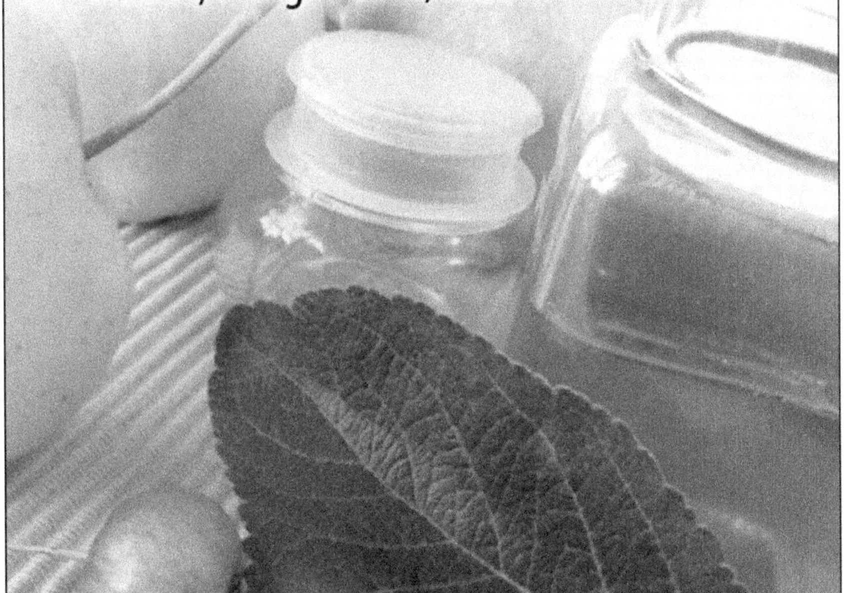

Table Of Contents

Introduction

I want to thank you and congratulate you for purchasing the book, *"Apple Cider Vinegar for Beginners: Proven Secrets Using Apple Cider Vinegar for Health, Weight Loss, Skin and Hair Care".*

This book contains proven steps and strategies on how to use apple cider vinegar to the fullest. This all-organic vinegar is pretty much effective for anything – for your skin, your hair, and your health.

Read on to know more about apple cider vinegar, how it is made, and why it is praised by millions of individuals worldwide.

Thanks again for purchasing this book, I hope you enjoy it!

Chapter 1: What is Apple Cider Vinegar?

In this age of modern medicine and technology, it is surprising to know that lots of people are interested about apple cider vinegar and actually using it. But what is apple cider vinegar? Is it really beneficial or just all hype?

Apple Cider Vinegar

Also known as ACV or cider vinegar, apple cider vinegar is a type of vinegar that's made from apples. Its color ranges from pale amber to medium yellowish-brown. While apple cider vinegar is clear, the organic and unpasteurized kind is foggy and slightly congealed. This is because of the large amounts of mother of vinegar in the ACV. Mother of vinegar is actually cellulose, a natural carbohydrate, that's produced by bacteria in the vinegar. It is not harmful when ingested or is it a sign of spoilage. It is actually what frequent ACV users look for.

How is it Made?

Apple cider vinegar is best used and consumed when unpasteurized, unfiltered, and organic. While this ACV type is readily available in stores, most individuals prefer to make it themselves. The overall process of making apple cider vinegar at home is easy albeit lengthy. Fermentation of ten takes about two to three months. The advantage about making your own ACV is that it is practically for free. This is because you don't need to buy whole apples or additional ingredients. You can use the apple cores, peels, and bits instead of throwing them out.

Here's how you can make your own apple cider vinegar:

From Apple Scraps

1 cup browned apple scraps (cores, peels, and bits) from organic apples

2 tablespoons sugar or raw honey

Chlorine-free water

Very clean wide mouth glass jar

1. Put all the apple scraps inside the glass jar. Top off the jar with water. Make sure that the scraps are completely submerged. You may also put a smaller jar on top of the bigger jar to prevent the scraps from floating up.

2. Cover jar with a clean piece of cloth or towel and hide away in a dark, warm place to ferment.

3. After a few days, the jar's contents should thicken with the presence of sediments and "the mother". You also will notice a lot of scum formation on top. Just spoon off the scum and mix the liquid before covering it again. Continue doing this for four weeks.

4. After a month of fermentation, begin tasting your homemade ACV. If the taste is strong enough for you, strain the liquid and transfer into a clean jar or bottle. Discard the apple scraps and place your vinegar in the fridge to stop the fermentation process.

Whole Apples

6 organic apples

2 teaspoons raw honey

2 teaspoons unpasteurized apple cider vinegar (optional)

Chlorine-free water

Large wide mouth jar or bowl

1. Cut the apple into quarters. Let them brown slightly. Place them in the jar or bowl.

2. Add the honey and, if using, unpasteurized apple cider vinegar too. Mix and cover the apples entirely with water. Cover the jar or bowl with a clean piece of cloth or cheesecloth.

3. Put in a warm, dark place for 6 months.

4. After the appropriate time, spoon off the scum formation on top. If you'll be making another batch of apple cider vinegar, remove the solid "mother" or the white film on top of the liquid and add it to the set of ingredients.

5. Taste the vinegar everyday if it is strong enough to your liking.

6. Strain the liquid and transfer it to another clean container. Cover with the clean piece of cloth for another month before bottling and storing in the fridge.

Things to Remember

1. Avoid using any metal containers or tools when making and storing apple cider vinegar. Utilize only plastic, wood, or glass.

2. Make sure that you store your apple cider vinegar in a place with a temperature of about 60 to 80 degrees Fahrenheit. Storing it in a lower or higher temperature would prevent fermentation.

3. Commit to stirring and shaking your apple cider everyday. If you fail to stir it, it would not turn into vinegar due to lack of oxygen.

Uses of Apple Cider Vinegar

Apple cider vinegar is often used by individuals as an ingredient when making vinaigrettes, chutneys, marinades, salad dressings, and more. But it is long been used as a miracle tonic too. As early as 1950's, apple cider vinegar allegedly treats myriad illnesses and conditions, detoxify the body from toxins, stop aging, and clean the entire house among others. While these claims lack scientific evidences, a lot of individuals and some doctors swear by apple cider vinegar's versatility and efficacy. In fact, the popularity of ACV has reached new heights this year. If you want to use this so-called miracle liquid other than an ingredient in your meal, proceed to the other chapters in this ebook to learn more.

Chapter 2: Apple Cider Vinegar for Health

Apple cider vinegar's health benefits are vast and many. It is not only used to cure trivial symptoms but is also used to combat more serious and fatal health problems too.

According to some people, the potency of apple cider vinegar is said to be because of its high acetic acid concentration. If frequently consumed, the acetic acid can increase the body's capability to absorb vitamins and minerals from the food that you eat. Apple cider vinegar is also rich in enzymes, potassium, and other organic acids like propionic acid and lactic acid. This supposedly explains why ACV drinkers feel healthier.

Apart from these, here are other explanations why apple cider vinegar is good for you:

Lowers Cholesterol

The high concentration level of acetic acid and potassium in apple cider vinegar is said to lower bad cholesterol level in the body. These components are said to thin the blood to allow it to flow and circulate properly. Although more research is needed to back up this claim, some individuals have said that their cholesterol level have in fact decreased after a month of taking ½ ounce of apple cider vinegar daily.

Controls Blood Sugar

Ingesting two tablespoons of apple cider vinegar before bed or before every meal helps lower the blood sugar and glucose level of people with type 2 diabetes by 4% to 6%. While more research is needed to solidly attest this finding, individuals who suffer from diabetes who routinely take ACV daily confirmed this decrease.

Decongests Stuffy Nose

If you are suffering from nasal congestion, drink a glass of water mixed with a tablespoon of apple cider vinegar to get relief. The potassium and acetic acid in the vinegar effectively stops bacteria growth in the sinus while simultaneously thinning out mucus.

Stops Hiccups

Annoying hiccups don't stand a chance with a teaspoonful of tangy apple cider vinegar. The sour taste of the liquid will overwhelm the nerves in the throat, causing it to relax and cease the hiccup attack.

Prevents Indigestion

Stuffing yourself with good food may seem to be a good idea but that was before you suffered from indigestion. The next time you head out to for the buffet, make sure to drink a concoction made from a teaspoon each of honey and apple cider vinegar and 8 ounces of water. To be taken 20 to 30 minutes before a meal, this ACV mixture will help prevent heartburn, stomach cramps, acid reflux, nausea, and other symptoms of indigestion.

Cures Sore Throat

Bacteria and germs that cause sore throat cannot survive in an acidic environment. If you are experiencing the beginning symptoms of a sore throat, fight off the infection by gargling a mixture of ¼ cup apple cider vinegar and warm water every hour.

Relieves Leg Cramps

Leg cramps are due to the lack of potassium in the body. This can be corrected by drinking a mixture of one tablespoon of honey, two tablespoons apple cider vinegar, and 8 ounces of water. If you are prone to leg cramps, have this concoction handy and consume whenever it occurs to immediately put a stop to your suffering.

Stops Stomach Woes

If you are suffering from diarrhea, spasms, and other stomach problems, drink two tablespoons of apple cider vinegar that's mixed in a glass of clear juice or water. The antibiotic properties of the ACV halt any bacterial infections while the pectin in the vinegar effectively soothes the pain.

Eases Asthma

While it is not a substitute for asthma spray and medication, apple cider vinegar contains properties that helps relaxes the throat to make breathing easier during an attack.

Sustains Bone Mass

Consuming apple cider vinegar daily discharges calcium and other bone-building minerals from the food to ensure that it is absorbed quickly and more efficiently by the body. Some studies show that individuals who religiously drink ACV actually absorb one-thirds more than those who didn't. Of course, it doesn't hurt that apple cider vinegar is also rich in calcium.

Fights Candida (Yeast Overgrowth)

The acids and enzyme in the apple cider vinegar kills excess yeast found in the body. Drinking one tablespoon daily of this miracle liquid on an empty stomach can flush out the toxins. If you experience worsening of the symptoms upon initial ACV intake, don't be alarmed. This just means that your body isn't removing the toxins fast enough. Continue taking the ACV and soon your body will purge all the yeast out. You may also soak in a tub filled with warm water and 1 ½ cups of ACV for about 20 minutes if you can't stomach the taste of apple cider vinegar.

Stops Exhaustion

Stress and intense exercise can cause exhaustion and fatigue. The potassium and various enzymes found in apple cider vinegar eliminate lactic acid build-up in the body to ensure a steady stream of energy. Make an extra refreshing energy drink by adding two tablespoons of apple cider vinegar to one glass of chilled tomato or carrot juice.

Relieves Arthritis and Joint Pain

Arthritis and other diseases which cause joint stiffness and pains are caused by mineral deficiency as well as toxin crystal buildup in the joints. Incessant intake of apple cider vinegar prevents this mineral shortage because it is rich in potassium, magnesium, phosphorus, and calcium. Also, the pectin in ACV absorbs the toxins and flushes them out before they accumulate in the joints. Apart from drinking the apple cider vinegar, it can be applied directly on the aching joint. Mix two tablespoons ACV to one tablespoon virgin coconut oil and massage on the affected area for relief. Soaking your aching feet or hands for several minutes in six cups of warm water and one cup of ACV also helps reduce the pain.

Chapter 3: Apple Cider Vinegar and Weight Loss

One of the main reasons why apple cider vinegar's popularity skyrocketed is because of many individuals' claim to weight loss. By just drinking two tablespoons of this miracle vinegar before meals daily, one could lose about ten to fifteen pounds in one year. But why is this possible? What does apple cider vinegar possesses that makes an individual lose weight?

Pectin

Apple cider vinegar is rich in complex carbohydrate called pectin. Pectin is a natural-occurring thickening agent that expands in the stomach when mixed with water. This helps make the person more satisfied and feel fuller longer after a meal. Pectin also aids in controlling cravings

Potassium

If a person eats too much salty food, his body will retain water so his weight will naturally go up. Apple cider vinegar prevents water retention because of high potassium content which effectively flushes sodium out of the body. With less retained water in the body, body weight would significantly decrease.

Acetic Acid

Apple cider vinegar's main component is acetic acid. This acid, when mixed with food, encourages higher protein absorption. The more protein the body absorbs, the higher the rate of oxygen utilization which leads to metabolic rate increase. A person who has high metabolic rate burns thrice as much calorie when engaging in daily activities, performing strenuous exercise, and even while at rest. The more calories burned, the more pounds lost.

Additional Functions of Apple Cider Vinegar

1. A naturally potent remedy for irritable bowel movement and diarrhea, apple cider vinegar stimulates and assists in digestion. It hastens removal of nutrients in the swallowed food for absorption and pushes the unwanted fat out from the intestines. This quick removal of fat avoids absorption to the body and prevents weight gain.

2. Apple cider vinegar releases huge amounts of tryptophan. This is an amino acid that's released from proteins during digestion. In turn, tryptophan releases serotonin which aids in relaxing the mind and the body to prevent stress eating.

3. Drinking apple cider vinegar daily maintains healthy alkaline pH level in the body. With a normal pH level, the body will be more energetic and can sustain intense bouts of exercise.

The weight loss of 15 pounds a year can be really trivial especially for very overweight people. To make significant progress in your aim to reach a healthy way, supplement your apple cider vinegar intake with lifestyle changes. This includes elimination of bad fat and excess sugar in the diet, and consumption of more fresh fruits, vegetables, and water. Of course, being in constant motion helps a lot in shedding unwanted body fat. You don't need to engage in really strenuous exercises. Low impact and enjoyable activities such as walking, swimming, biking, and various sports do great wonders for weight loss too.

Chapter 4: Apple Cider Vinegar and Detoxification

From the food that we eat, water we drink, and to the air that we breathe, the chances of toxin exposure is always high. In order to be healthier, undergoing a safe but effective detoxification process is strongly recommended.

Detoxification, or detox as many celebrities call it, is a process that is intended to flush out the toxins from the body. There are many detoxification methods to choose from to date. But the most popular one has to be the apple cider vinegar detox.

Just like what its name denotes, the apple cider vinegar detox uses apple cider vinegar to rid the body of harmful and illness-causing toxins. It is safe, natural, and possesses zero side effects. Apple cider vinegar is also rich in vitamins, minerals, and natural enzymes so your body won't feel deprived and weak even during the process of cleansing and purging.

Apple cider vinegar's potent components cleanse the lymph nodes by dissolving mucus found in the body. When the nodes are clear and have improved circulation, it can easily purge expel toxins that had accumulated in the cells. A healthy lymphatic system also reduces allergies, sinus infections, and mucous congestions.

Consuming apple cider vinegar daily encourages digestion and improves overall gastric health. If food is digested thoroughly, nutrients are absorbed faster and the waste and toxins are eliminated quickly before they have sufficient time to cause damage.

Apple Cider Vinegar Detox

Detoxification by way of apple cider vinegar intake is easy. But to ensure that you get real results, you should only use the best apple cider vinegar type. The apple cider vinegar that you should use must be the organic, raw, unprocessed, and unfiltered type. This type of ACV contains a lot of "mother" and makes all the difference. If you use another type of ACV, the detoxification process will be less effective or may not provide any advantages.

Apart from using drinking two tablespoons of apple cider vinegar daily, you should also consume other food and drinks that utilize apple cider vinegar as an ingredient. Continuous consumption and use of apple cider vinegar ensures total toxin flush.

ACV Detox Tea Drink

Ingredients: 2 tablespoons apple cider vinegar, 2 tablespoons lemon juice, 12 ounces filtered water (room temperature), 1 teaspoon cinnamon, a dash of cayenne pepper, and Stevia powder to taste

Directions: Mix all the ingredients together and consume immediately. Drink thrice a day for best results.

If you need a break from the taste of apple cider vinegar, you may choose to detoxify through soaking:

ACV Detox Bath

Draw a hot bath and add in 1 cup of Epsom salts and 1 cup of apple cider vinegar. Soak for a 20-30 minutes to draw out toxins from the skin, relieve aching joints, and heal acne or eczema.

Chapter 5: Apple Cider Vinegar and Skin Care

You might think that it's weird or gross to put a meal ingredient on your skin especially if it is something that has a really strong odor like apple cider vinegar. But a lot of women have ignored the smell because of ACV's potency to heal and improve skin's condition.

When applied, the components of apple cider vinegar improve blood circulation in the skin's small capillaries. The constant flow of blood frees any impurities to make the skin clearer and rosier. Apple cider vinegar is also antiseptic which helps heal and prevent acne and bacterial infections on the skin. The acetic acid found in the ACV balances the pH level of the skin. This helps lessen and prevent acne breakouts, excessive oil production, and skin scaling or peeling. The alpha hydroxyl acids in the apple cider vinegar also eliminate dead skin cells to show off a fresher and younger skin underneath.

Here are some ACV skin care recipes you can follow to have clearer, smoother, more beautiful skin:

ACV Facial Wash

In a small bowl, combine 6 tablespoons of warm water and 2 tablespoons of apple cider vinegar. For sensitive skin, start with 10 tablespoons of water to 2 tablespoons of apple cider vinegar. After washing your face with warm water, dip a cotton ball into the mixture and apply it on your face and neck using a gentle, upward motion. Continue cleaning your face until the cotton is free of dirt. Leave on the ACV wash for 15 minutes before rinsing. If the smell is tolerable, skip the rinse and apply a moisturizer straight after.

Herbal ACV Wash

Apple cider vinegar's potency triples when mixed with different herbs like lavender, rosemary, rosewood, and more. This is because these plants contain essential oils that aid in improving the skin's health and appearance.

Ingredients: Two pints apple cider vinegar, 3 ounces of elder flowers, and 2 ounces of calendula

OR

Two pints apple cider vinegar, and 1 ounce each lavender, linden flowers, and rose petals

Directions: Using a jar with lid, soak the plant materials in the apple cider vinegar. Secure the lid tightly. Place in a warm, bright place and allow the plant materials to macerate for two weeks. Strain and store in a clean bottle.

To use: add one tablespoon of the concoction to a cup of spring water to use as a facial wash or 5 tablespoons to a tub full of water to use as a bath soak.

In case you have essential oils on hand, you may also create this recipe:

Ingredients: 3/5 teaspoon rosemary essential oil, 3/5 teaspoon lavender essential oil, 2/5 teaspoon rosewood essential oil, 1 cup filtered water, 17 ½ fluid ounce apple cider vinegar and 2 tablespoons glycerin

Directions: Mix all the ingredients together. Soak a cotton ball in the mixture and dab all over the face. Let dry before rinsing.

pH Balancing Toner

This balancing toner will help ward off pimple-causing bacteria, shed dead skin cells, and unblock pores.

Ingredients: 2 cups distilled water and ½ cup apple cider vinegar

*always shake well before using

Directions: Combine the two ingredients and put inside a clean and sterilized glass bottle. Apply the toner on clean skin using a cotton ball or pad. Leave to dry on the skin and rinse well. Follow with a moisturizer immediately. For use on the body, place on a spray bottle and spritz on back acne or blackheads.

Pepper-Rose Toner

Brighten your skin, reduce itchiness, and control excess oil with this peppermint and rosemary toner.

Ingredients: 2 tablespoons apple cider vinegar, 8 drops peppermint essential oil, 10 drops rosemary essential oil, and 1 cup filtered or distilled water

Directions: Combine all the ingredients in a glass bottle. Shake well. Apply on skin daily. If you find the toner too drying, reduce the apple cider vinegar to 1 tablespoon.

Detox Face Mask

Remove deep seated dirt and open up clogged pores with this cleansing mask:

Ingredients: bentonite clay, apple cider vinegar, and 1 tablespoon raw honey.

Directions: Mix equal parts of bentonite clay and apple cider vinegar in a bowl. Add the honey and stir well. Apply on clean face and leave on for 15 minutes. Rinse with warm water.

Age-Spot Reducer

Target age spots and reduce their appearance with this toner:

Ingredients: 2 tablespoons apple cider vinegar and 1 tablespoon orange juice

Directions: Mix both ingredients well. Soak a cotton ball to the mixture and spot treat age spots. Leave on overnight.

OR

Ingredients: ¼ cup fresh onion juice (made from raw onion) and ¼ cup apple cider vinegar

Directions: Mix the ingredients in a small bowl and apply on face twice daily. You might want to wear goggles during application. Leave on overnight.

DIY Skin Brightener

This skin brightener gently exfoliates skin, removes excess oil, and provides a natural glow. It also reduces swelling and redness caused by acne.

Ingredients: 3 ounces distilled water, ½ ounce apple cider vinegar, and 5 pieces uncoated, plain aspirin tablets

Directions: Mix the water and apple cider vinegar in a bowl. Set aside. Crush the aspirin tablets into a fine powder using a pestle or mortar. Add it to the ACV mixture. Stir well to dissolve the powder. Apply the toner on the face weekly.

Herbal Moisturizing Spritz (for sensitive skin)

Mix 1 part apple cider vinegar, 4 parts green tea, and 3 drops Argan oil. Transfer in a spray bottle and spritz on face when needed. Shake well before use.

Sunburn Reliever

Relieve sunburn pain and prevent peeling and blistering with this ACV soak:

Add one cup of apple cider vinegar to your warm bath and soak for 8 to 10 minutes. The initial dip might sting a bit but will subside after a few minutes.

Wart Removal

Crush ½ garlic clove and place directly on the wart. Soak a bandage in pure apple cider vinegar and use it to wrap the wart overnight. By morning, remove the bandage and rinse the wart in cold water. Generously apply castor oil on the wart and cover with a dry bandage. Continue the night and morning bandage wrap routine until the wart effortlessly falls off.

Callus Removal

Completely soak the hand or foot in undiluted apple cider vinegar for 30 minutes up to 1 hour. Use a pumice stone to trim off the hardened skin. Soak the affected area again for 15 minutes and rinse. Repeat weekly.

Athlete's Foot Relief

Eliminate foot odor and itching brought upon by athlete's foot by soaking your feet in a concoction made with equal parts apple cider vinegar and water. If you want a stronger mix, add 1/3 cup of Listerine mouthwash (original variant).

Chapter 6: Apple Cider Vinegar for Hair Care

A true miracle liquid, apple cider vinegar does wonders to the hair and scalp too. It cleanses the hair and adds the much needed body and luster. If you are experiencing hair loss, itchy scalp, and dandruff, you'll be glad to know that apple cider vinegar can effectively provide remedies for them too.

ACV Hair Conditioner

Ingredients: apple cider vinegar and filtered water

Directions: Combine 1 part apple cider vinegar to 4 parts water. Transfer to a spray bottle and mix well. Squeeze out excess water from your wet hair. Separate your hair into sections and liberally spray the ACV conditioner on the scalp and hair from roots to tips. Massage in the conditioner and let sit for a few minutes. Rinse with water.

*the smell of this ACV conditioner may be too potent for some. If it bothers you, use it only when you are staying in at home.

Cold Hair Rinse

Ingredients: 1 cup apple cider vinegar and 16 ounces water

Directions: Mix the ACV and water. Place in a bottle and store in the fridge to cool. To use, apply the vinegar rinse after shampooing the hair.

Herb Vinegar Rinse

Ingredients: 2 tablespoons of appropriate *dried herb, 1 pint water, and 1 pint of apple cider vinegar

*herbs:

For dark hair: rosemary

For light hair: chamomile

For dry hair: marigold

For brittle hair: horsetail

For oily hair: thyme

Directions:

Grab a tea ball and put in two tablespoons of the dried herb of your choice. Let it steep in a pint of freshly boiled water for two hours. Once cool, transfer the infusion in a sizeable jar and add in the apple cider vinegar. Mix well. Pour the rinse on newly washed hair and massage for a few minutes.

EO Hair Rinse

Ingredients: 5 drops of sage or rose essential oil, 1 cup warm water, and 1 cup apple cider vinegar

Directions: Add the essential oil to the ACV and stir. To use: take one tablespoon of the essential oil mix and combine to a cup of warm water. Pour on the hair and leave on for several minutes before rinsing.

ACV and Herb Rinse (for damaged or thinning hair)

Ingredients: 3 tablespoons of dried hops, 2 tablespoons of apple cider vinegar, and 2 cups of water.

Directions: Using a saucepan, allow the water to boil. Lower the heat and let simmer. Add the vinegar and herbs. Do not stir. Cover the pan and let the herb steep for 15 minutes. Remove from heat, strain the liquid, and let cool.

To use: Apply the rinse after shampooing the hair. Massage into the scalp for several minutes. Avoid getting the rinse in your eyes. Rinse out with plain water.

Itchy Scalp and Dandruff Relief

Apply undiluted apple cider vinegar to your dry scalp and hair and massage for several minutes. Leave on for one hour before rinsing.

Thinning Hair

Stir in a pinch of cayenne powder to 2 tablespoons of apple cider vinegar. Rub it on the affected area before showering. Rinse well.

Bald Spots

Pierce 1 royal jelly capsule and squeeze out its content in a small bowl. Add one teaspoon of apple cider vinegar and mix well. Pat on bald spots and leave overnight. Rinse as usual.

Product Build-Up Remover

Ingredients: apple cider vinegar, lemon juice, and water

Directions: Mix 1 part apple cider vinegar and 2 parts water. Add in 2-3 tablespoons of lemon juice and stir. Transfer in a spray bottle and shake well. Spray on clean hair and leave on until dry.

Natural Hair Lice Remover

Ingredients: lavender essential oil, olive oil, 1 tablespoon apple cider vinegar and 1 cup water.

Directions: Combine 1 part lavender essential oil to 3 parts olive oil. Completely saturate the hair and scalp with this oil mixture and cover with a shower cap for 5 hours. Mix the apple cider vinegar and water and use this to rinse the oil off. Remove the lice and nits using a very fine-tooth comb. Repeat the process every other day up to 10 days until the lice are completely eradicated.

Conclusion

Thank you again for purchasing this book!

I hope this book was able to help you to appreciate the natural wonder that is apple cider vinegar.

The next step is to try the appropriate remedies that apple cider vinegar has to offer you. You have absolutely nothing to lose and everything to gain. Join the millions of people who had found relief by using ACV.

Finally, if you enjoyed this book, please take the time to share your thoughts and post a review on Amazon. We do our best to reach out to readers and provide the best value we can. Your positive review will help us achieve that. It'd be greatly appreciated!

Thank you and good luck!

Book 3:

Body Butters For Beginners:

BY LINDSEY P

Proven Secrets To Making All Natural Body Butters For Rejuvenating And Hydrating Your Skin

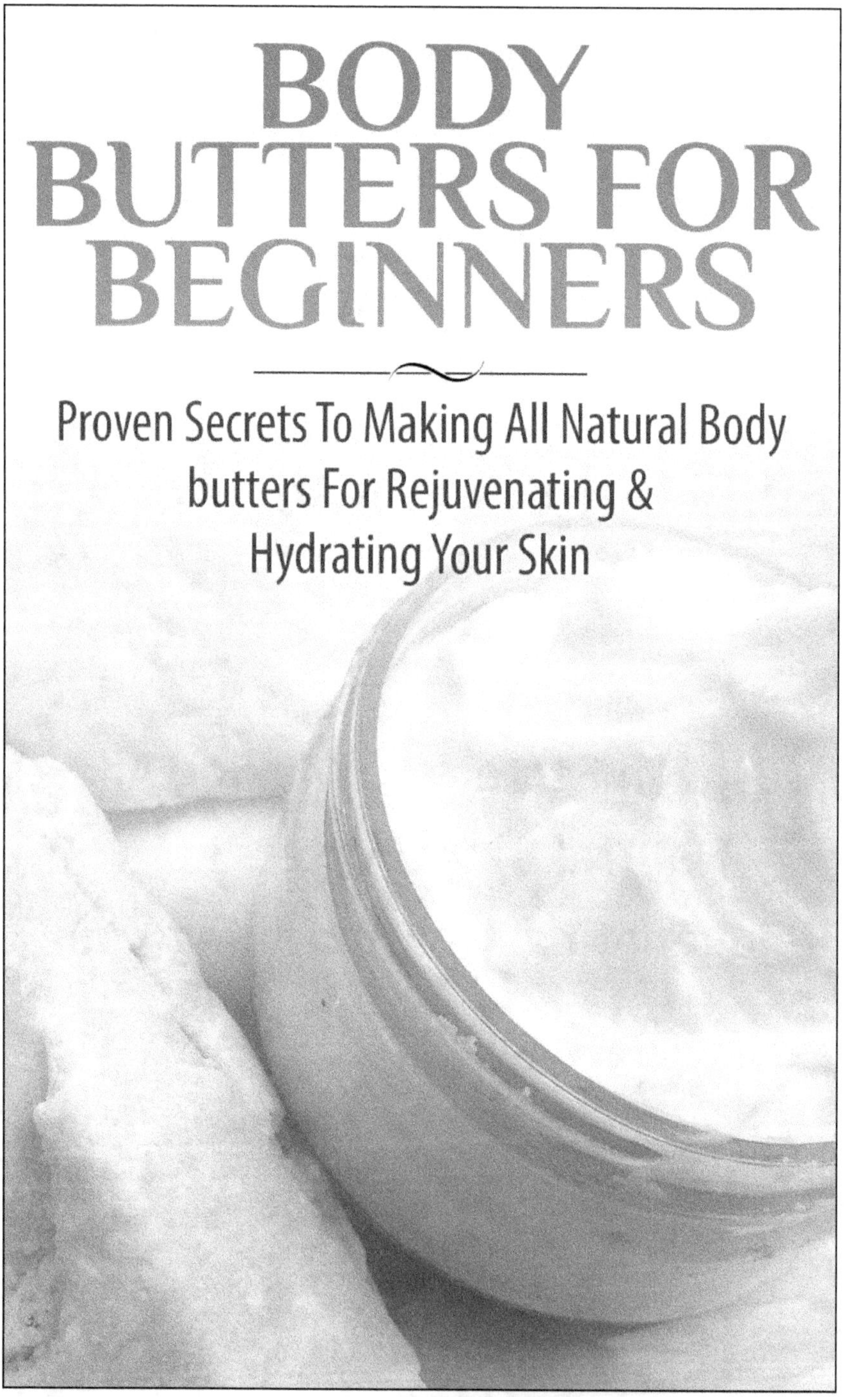

BODY BUTTERS FOR BEGINNERS

Proven Secrets To Making All Natural Body butters For Rejuvenating & Hydrating Your Skin

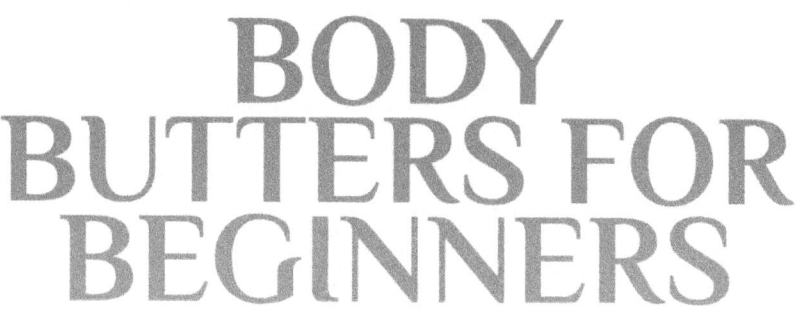

Table Of Contents

Introduction

I want to thank you and congratulate you for purchasing the book, *"Body Butters For Beginners: Proven Secrets To Making All Natural Body Butters For Rejuvenating And Hydrating Your Skin"*
This book contains proven steps and strategies on how to have radiant and healthy skin with the help of body butters, which you can make all by yourself and at the comfort of your home.

Do you know that having healthy and beautiful skin is as easy as ABC? With simple to follow steps, you can make your own body butters! Whether you are a beginner or an expert chef, you can dish out a body butter recipe for you and your loved ones – not to be eaten of course, but to be applied on the skin. Say goodbye to dry, scaly skin and start giving your skin the star treatment it deserves.

Thanks again for purchasing this book, I hope you enjoy it!

Chapter 1 Deeper Than Skin Deep

Deeper Than Skin Deep

Healthy skin equals a healthy you

Beautiful skin makes all the difference when it comes to total physical beauty. How could it not? The skin is the largest organ of the body and you simply can't avoid seeing it.

When you see famous celebrities in movies and on TV, the first thing you would usually notice about them is their flawless skin. These stars know the importance of taking care of their skin. It is not just superficial for them.

The care for the skin is from inside out. Well, you are a star in your own right and your skin deserves that star treatment as well. You would not regret all the time and finances you spend on taking care of your skin. It would glow and people would know. A healthy skin is something you cannot hide.

How does one achieve an overall great and healthy skin? First, get to know the skin very well. What is it? What is it made of? What does it need?

Your first line of defense

Skin is very important in protecting you and everything inside your body. Imagine, if you do not have skin? It would be gross to see the muscles, bones, and organs all out, wouldn't it? And you would not last long what with all the foreign bodies and infections that might set in to your vital organs.

You could really say that the value of skin is really more than skin deep. It's technically life for everybody. Not only does it protect your body, it also helps your body maintain the right temperature. And without skin how would you be able to feel that tender touch of your loved ones?

Nobody can boast that he or she would survive without the help of the skin. So, maintaining it to be healthy is a must for all. This is, after all, your first line of defense against whatever is the enemy of the body.

What is skin made of? Let's find out.

Parts of skin: three layers

1. Epidermis – the outermost layer. This is what you can see and touch. If you look at the skin on your hand right now, it seems like nothing is going on in there, right? Do not be deceived. Just beneath it is a busy network of different cells and organisms with the sole purpose of making new skin cells. After 2 weeks or a month, these new skin cells would move up to the epidermis. As new cells arise, the old ones die and move on top of the epidermis where they would be shed off. Around 30k-40k of dead cells are being shed off every minute! Imagine, just by reading this alone, millions of cells have died and have been replaced already in your body. Could the body catch up on replacing these with new cells? You need not worry as the epidermis works 95% all the time to make new skin for you. The other 5% works for melanin. This gives the color of your skin. The darker you are, the more melanin is produced. This keeps you safe from the sun's harmful rays. They make extra melanin to protect you from being sunburned. However, your skin cannot do it alone. It needs you to help protect

itself from the destructive effects of the sun. You can do this by applying sunblock or using an umbrella or wearing a hat during a sunny day.

2. Dermis – lies just beneath the epidermis. This is where the blood vessels, nerves, sweat and oil glands are located. There is where you'll find the tough and stretchy collagen and elastin. Nerve endings help you to feel – whether what you have touched was hot or cold. The blood vessels deliver and supply nutrients and oxygen to the skin. Oil or sebaceous glands produce the skin's natural oil called sebum. This body's oil protects and lubricates the skin. Sebum acts as the body's waterproof shield. Have you seen water and oil mix? Sebum makes sure you won't absorb so much water that your skin would be soggy. Sweat glands protect the skin too. They came through pores or the tiny holes in the skin.

3. Subcutaneous fat –the bottom part of the skin, which is mostly made of fat. It helps the body to be warm. It also absorbs shock if you fall down or hit something. This is where the hair follicles are located, too.

Functions of the skin

As you know by now, your skin protects the whole body. It also warms or cools you so that you maintain 37 degrees C or 98.6 degrees F which is the ideal temperature for the body. During a hot day, your body would release heat through the skin to cool you down. So you perspire a lot. When it is cold, your body would preserve heat to keep you warm.

The skin is really deeper than skin deep. It deserves special attention and care. There are many products that can help you moisturize and keep your skin healthy, supple and glowing. Learn more about them as you read on.

Chapter 2 Which Is Which?

Which is which?

Skin care and skin products flood the market. This is a growing industry, which is getting and getting more popular as the years pass. The consumers are sometimes confused which products would benefit them the most.

A lot of people are willing to spend so much just to have beautiful skin. They sometimes commit the error of just buying the most expensive product. Price is not necessarily the basis of how good a skin product is for your skin.

To get the most out of these skin products, you should first know your skin type. There are different skin types. The factors that may affect your skin type include the race, age, weather or season and your overall health status. If you cannot personally determine your skin type, then you can avail the help of the professionals. Your skin is worth it.

Assess your skin type.

There are four skin types– dry, oily, normal and combination.

- Dry skin - this is medically termed as xeroderma. This is due to lack of water on the epidermis. As one ages too, the amount of natural oils and lubricants also diminish which lead to dry skin. The body parts prone to dryness are the arms, elbows, knees, and the lower legs. Aside from ageing, the other causes of dry skin are harsh soaps and other skin products, extreme weather, poor water intake and hot showers.

- Oily skin – the body produces natural oils. For some reasons, some people produce more body oil than what is needed. The following are the possible causes of your oily skin: genes (it runs in your family), overuse of skin products, weather conditions, some drugs, and stress. Oily skin causes acne and skin breakouts. Toners, cleansers, blotting papers and medicated pads are used to manage excessive oily skin.
- Normal skin – some people cannot distinguish if they have normal skin. That is because sometimes, the skin appears oily one time and dry the next. A normal skin has no trace of oil. It feels supple and elastic. And it has the least problem when it comes to skin conditions.
- Combination–this is common and in the face, it could be that some parts are oily (usually the nose and forehead) and some are dry, like the cheeks.

Various skin products

Now that you are aware of the type of skin that you have, you go to the next step. Determine which product your skin needs. You are already aware that your skin's primary need is hydration. There are different hydration elements. The two most common are humectant and lubricant.

- Humectant –these retain or preserve the moisture
- Lubricant – "trap" moisture or prevent it from escaping, serving as a barrier to the skin

While both lotions and moisturizers possess these elements, not all products containing these would automatically make your skin healthy. Lotions are less viscous, meaning they are more fluid-like and thinner. They have lighter consistency. This is why they are usually in a container where you can pump it.

Lotions can retain moisture that is already within the skin but not as much. They have less oil content so they do not lubricate well. For normal skin, these products would suffice.

However, for drier skin, you would need added protection and moisture-retaining products. For those individuals who have extra-dry skin, even the strongest lotion would not be enough to combat the dryness. You might want to consider trying body butters.

Know more about this skin wonder product as you read on.

Chapter 3 Discovering Body Butters

Discovering Body Butters

What are body butters?

You may not be aware of body butters. These are actually moisturizers that contain lubricating ingredients. They are technically like lotions, only better. These ingredients serve as a protective barrier or a shield so that moisture would stay within the skin and outside environmental elements that may be harmful to the skin would not be able to come in.

Body butters are more emollient, have high viscosity and more effective for those with dry skin. Some examples of these lubricating ingredients are shea butter, coconut oil, olive and jojoba oils. Consumers also describe body butters as ensuring a "more luxurious" feel on their skin.

Body butters are extra moisturizing because they contain less water and have more essential oils or butters needed by the body to maintain moisture. Viscosity and consistency are greater so these butters are placed in jars where they would be scooped, because it would be difficult to pump them out.

Another wonder of body butter is it is ideal for those with sensitive skin. Allergies or rashes seldom occur because the ingredients of body butters are all-natural. Usually, a body butter is made up of an oil base and a few more ingredients. You would appreciate the fact that they are free from various chemicals and preservatives that could harm your skin.

Do you want to know another wonder of body butters? You could actually make your own right at the comfort of your home. They are easy to make and the ingredients are not hard to find, too.

Are you ready for a healthier skin? Find out more about making your own body butters.

Chapter 4 Beauty Within Your Reach

Beauty Within Your Reach

It is time to end the confusion on which products suit you. It is time to make your own body butters.

One great thing about body butters is the availability of the ingredients. You could avail of these even from your local stores. You would notice though that the ingredients are mostly derived from nuts and seeds. So if you have allergies to these, it is wise to consult your primary health care provider first just to be sure if topical applications would be hazardous to you.

Here are some of the basic ingredients of body butter.

1. Cocoa butter – Cocoa butter is made from cocoa beans. Cocoa beans come from the fleshy cocoa fruits. After cleaning and roasting, the beans are placed in a machine where the cocoa butter would be produced. Of course, in your local store, you could just buy it as a cocoa butter already. This is actually a vegetable fat that is edible. It is used mostly for making chocolates and beauty products. What makes this as a good ingredient to help your skin? The cocoa itself contains large amounts of antioxidants called flavonoids. It is also rich in potassium, calcium and iron. These allow veins to be more relaxed. This promotes good circulation and at the same time, help fight against free radicals that are harmful to the body. Not to mention, this smells good too.

2. Shea butter – Another common ingredient of body butter is shea butter. This comes from the nut of the

African shea tree or karite tree. This is also known as karite butter. Like the cocoa butter, this extracted fat is also edible and can be used in making chocolates. This ingredient has been known to be very effective in the fight against stretch marks. It has been internationally recognized to treat various skin disorders as well. This is because it has been found to contain anti-inflammatory properties. It is also an anti-ageing agent. The vitamins found in shea butter help in preventing the occurrence of wrinkles and other facial lines. Plus it can be a form of sunblock and even as a relief for nasal congestion and sinusitis.

3. Coconut oil – Much has been written about the wonders of this ingredient. In some tropical areas, the coconut tree is considered as the tree of life. It has been used for thousands of years not only as skin beautifier but as supplements to help conquer Alzheimer disease, Diabetes Mellitus, Thyroid problems, weight concerns and even hair problems like lice and dandruff. Coconut is known to be the number one source of lauric acids. These acids have been known to fight off pathogens or harmful organisms in the body.

4. Mango butter – Another great ingredient is mango butter which is an oil extracted from the kernel of a mango. It has anti-inflammatory, anti-oxidant and anti-ageing properties, making it a favorite among cosmetics suppliers. It contains oleic and stearic acids in very large amounts. These make mango butter highly emollient and thus ideal in sealing moisture within the body. It highly

nourishes the skin, too. Plus it has a very sweet and refreshing smell. Mango butter can also provide protection from the sun. It also non-greasy and very soothing to touch.

5. Cinnamon – The common kitchen ingredient cinnamon has some uncommon qualities. Do you know that it is a proven antimicrobial, anti-fungal and antibacterial agent? What's more, it has an astringent property, which helps make the skin firmer and clearer as it removes blemishes. Cinnamon is gaining popularity because it is also very rich in magnesium, iron and calcium. These are minerals that help keep skin healthy. Cinnamon is great for body butters as it also helps local blood circulation. A good circulation allows for delivery of nutrients and oxygen to the different parts of the body. This has been used in the fight against acne and has shown to remove impurities and to aid as an anti inflammatory substance as well.

6. Honey – Raw honey is a humectant. It helps retain water so that the skin is kept moisturized. Honey as a cosmetic agent has been used for thousands of years already. It was discovered to contain skin restorative properties. Just a little amount can go a long way in making the skin youthful looking. Honey also contains germ-fighting bacteria, which help in fighting off the enemies of the skin.

7. Other ingredients – do not be surprise that other nuts and seeds can be included as ingredients too in any body butter that you could make. As long as there is the base oil or lubricant, you could add other ingredients that could enhance the feel, the smell and the color of the body butter. These are peppermint, rosemary, lavender, magnesium, black raspberry, coffee, cinnamon, vanilla, lemon, avocado and the list goes on.

You can enjoy tremendous peace of mind since you are 100% sure that what you are using won't harm your skin or make it look unsightly. With these ingredients, you could start making your own body butter now. Plus it can also be a great gift idea for your family and friends.

Having healthy skin need not be difficult nor expensive. Start having great skin that you could show off! Start making your own body butters.

Chapter 5 Simple Recipes For A Great Skin

Simple Recipes For Great Skin

Do you know that you can make as many as one hundred or more different body butters for your skin? That's right, and all these at the comfort of your own home with no special machinery needed. You do not even have to be a chef to do these. You could be a beginner and a master at making body butters at the same time.

Here are simple tips before you start.

1. Remember to check if you have any allergic reaction or even sensitivity to any of the ingredients that you are going to use. If unsure, it is better to try it out on a small portion of your arm first. If there are no untoward reactions, such as itchiness, redness, warm feeling or any sign of irritation, then you can try it on other parts until you have proven that it is safe for you.

2. Melting the oils is one basic action in making your own body butter. Try to melt it slowly by using low to medium level of heat. Do not place the oil at a high level of heat at any time.

3. You would also be asked to chill or set the oil. This is allowing the oils to cool and then form into a semi-solid state. If you would set it in a room temperature, it could take hours. In the refrigerator, estimated time for the oils to set is 15-20 minutes. Chilling properly is important because you would not want it to be frozen. It could kill some of the vitamins and minerals on the oils,

rendering it useless. And you would also have difficulty in getting the right viscosity of the body butter.

4. Finally, you would be asked to whip it until it reaches the butter-like consistency.

The body butters should be placed on clean glass jars.

The finished product should be maintained at a cool temperature to keep if from melting. However, if it melts, simply stir or whip it again until it returns to its previous consistency.

The homemade product's lifespan depends on many factors, but to be on the safe side, try to use it for three months at the most. There are reports of 6 months up to a year of useful life for these products.

Cooking Time

It is time to start making those body butters. Here are 10 simple recipes that you could use.

1. Triple delight body butter – Simply melt 1 cup shea butter and ½ cup coconut oil in the top of a double boiler. Once melted, allow the mixture to cool for 30 minutes. Stir in the half cup of almond oil. Place in the freezer or chiller (this is very important – chilling should just be right. It is about 20 minutes). Whip into a butter-like consistency when the oil starts to partially become solid. Place in a clean jar and then use for hydrating and rejuvenating your skin. Keep in a cool place. Simple right?

2. Vanilla Secret Body Butter – Do you know that vanilla can serve as aphrodisiac? Feel sexier as you use this body butter. Melt a cup of cocoa butter and half cup of coconut

oil. Remove from heat and allow to cool for thirty minutes. While waiting to cool, grind in a coffee grinder (or you could also use a food processor) a single vanilla bean. Place in a container. Stir in half cup of sweet almond oil into the vanilla bits plus the cooled oil mixture. Place in a freezer to chill. Wait until the oils start to be partially solid. Then using an electric mixer or a food processor, whip until it becomes like butter. There you have a vanilla body butter, which you could use to attract your partner too.

3. Mango & Shea Body Butter - Combine the following ingredients in a double boiler – ½ cup shea butter, ½ cup mango butter, ½ cup coconut oil and ½ cup olive or jojoba. Constantly stir as you melt all the oils. Remove from heat and allow to cool for 30 minutes. Place in the freezer until it starts to harden but it is still soft. Whip until fluffy and there you have it! Your own body butter for a more beautiful skin!

4. Rose Scented Coconut body butter – As you melt, cool and place the cup of coconut oil in the freezer, just add a few drops of rose scented oil to perfect the moisturizer. When in a semi solid stage, whip until it becomes butter-like in consistency. You would not only have a soft skin but you would simply adore that perfume like smell.

5. No-cook body butter – place all the ingredients in a food processor or blender. These are ¾ cup melted coconut oil, ½ tablespoons vanilla powder, ¼ cup cacao powder and 1/3 cup clear agave. Blend and then place them in clean glass or jars and then place in the refrigerator to set in.

6. Fruity body butter – combine half cup each of cocoa and shea butters. Melt and allow to cool. Add around 10-20 drops (depends on how fruity you like it to smell) of

Black Raspberry Fragrance Oil. Place in the refrigerator to set it. Once it is almost solid, whip it until it becomes like butter in consistency. You will then have a body butter that smells so cool.

7. Lemony Body Butters – Place 6 tablespoons coconut oil and ¼ cup cacao butter in a saucepan and melt it. Remove from heat and add 1 teaspoon lemon essential oil. Cool until the mixture solidifies. Whip and it is ready to use. You would love its refreshing lemon smell.

8. Pretty in Pink Body butter – this is a great idea for a gift. It looks charming with its pink color too. Melt 6 ounces coconut oil and 2 ounces cocoa butter in a low heat double boiler. After melting, remove from heat and let it cool. You could make this faster by placing it in the refrigerator. Once it is partially solid, you can whip this manually or use an electric mixer. The oils would turn creamy. Place this creamy oil in the refrigerator again for five minutes and then whip again. At this point, you could add essential oil like rosemary or peppermint until you get stiff peaks. As it is, it is already attractive and healthy for your skin. However, you could make it daintier by adding red colorant to the finished product, giving it a pinkish shade.

9. Glowing Skin Body Butter – the secret to this recipe is the use of extra virgin, raw and organic coconut oil. The feel afterwards is extra smooth and soft skin. Like the other recipes, just add this special 2 cups of coconut oil and 7 ounces of shea butter and allow to melt in a saucepan. Cool and at this time, you could add a drop of tea tree oil. Tea tree oil is known for its antimicrobial and antibacterial properties. You could also add any essential oils that you like. Peppermint, jasmine or rosemary smells great on this combination. This is

optional though. Cool, set in and then whip. You now have a body butter that is sure to make your skin healthier and softer.

10. Cinnamon Power Packed Body Butter – Melt 50 grams cocoa butter and 50 grams shea butter until it becomes a liquid. Add 100 grams coconut oil, stir in gently for a minute and then remove the oils from heat. Let it cool for 30 minutes. Add 30 drops of cinnamon oil as soon as it cools. Then whip until it becomes fluffy and butter-like. Before pouring it to containers, add some bits of cinnamon stick on it. Preferable containers are airtight.

That was easy, right? Even a first timer would get it right. You could do some mixing and matching of ingredients and you could even invent your own body butter. Make your own until you find the one that suits you perfectly. You would know if it is the perfect one for you when your skin feels so soft and smooth. You would also notice that your skin looks hydrated. This is because the moisture is locked in.

It is also recommended that you try and change the skin products every six months. This is to have a variety of available minerals and vitamins for your skin. Changing your body butters would also allow you to enjoy different smells and effects on your skin.

Chapter 6 More Tips For A Healthier Skin

More Tips For A Healthier Skin

Healthy Radiant Skin

Body butters and other moisturizers are big help when it comes to rejuvenated and hydrated skin. However, there are other things you could do to ensure a healthier skin.

Basic care for the skin

Caring for the skin cannot be overemphasized. Here are some simple things you can do to care for your skin.

1. Clean according to skin type. Different skin types require different kind of cleaning. For dry skin, use a mild cleansing product and clean only once, preferably at night. For oily skin, you could wash and clean it twice in a day. For the combination type, combine also the style of cleansing. For normal skin, regular washing would do. Follow the instructions on the labels of the products carefully.
2. Remove all make up. As much as possible, allow your skin to rest by not wearing any make up. If you do need to wear makeup, make sure that you totally remove it at the end of the day by washing thoroughly. Pat dry.
3. Protection from the sun. Your skin's number one enemy is the sun, although the sun is a friend from 7-8am. Afterwards, try to avoid its harmful rays as much as possible. You could apply sunscreen, use umbrella or wear clothes with sleeves.

4. Exfoliate. This simply means to remove the dead skin (you have millions of them remember?). You could do this on skin without breaks. There are products available in your local grocery store for exfoliation. Follow the instructions very well.

5. Water. When you think of skin, you want it to be hydrated at all times. By simply drinking 8-10 glasses a day, you are already helping your skin to be hydrated and radiant.

6. Do not scratch, pick on pimples, remove scabs or do anything that would break the skin. Keep it intact at all cost. You should also try to trim your nails so that they would not cause damage to your skin.

7. Supplements to help. Aside from eating healthy foods like fruits and vegetables, vitamins a, b, c and e can also help skin become healthier, softer and more beautiful.

8. Healthy lifestyle. Drinking alcoholic beverages, sleeping late, smoking, and eating junk foods are just some of the way that would harm your skin. Try having healthy habits and get enough rest and sleep.

9. Lotions and other products. To keep your skin from drying or just to moisturize it, there are various products that you can choose from and use. Find which one suits you best. Extreme weathers would require that you use these products more often to protect your skin.

A healthy skin is a goal that everybody must have. Skin care is easy and the rewards are awesome. Hydrated and rejuvenated skin looks great and at the same time, it is a great protector of the body. Enjoy a smooth and flawless skin now!

Conclusion

Thank you again for purchasing this book!

I hope this book was able to help you to start having great skin with very little efforts and cost by making your all-natural, easy to make body butters.

The next step is to enjoy that flawless and smooth skin. Share the secret to others too, by sharing this book to them.

Finally, if you enjoyed this book, please take the time to share your thoughts and post a review on Amazon. We do our best to reach out to readers and provide the best value we can. Your positive review will help us achieve that. It'd be greatly appreciated!

Thank you and good luck!

Book 4:

Coconut Oil for Easy Weight Loss

BY LINDSEY P

A Step by Step Guide for Using Virgin Coconut Oil for Quick and Easy Weight Loss

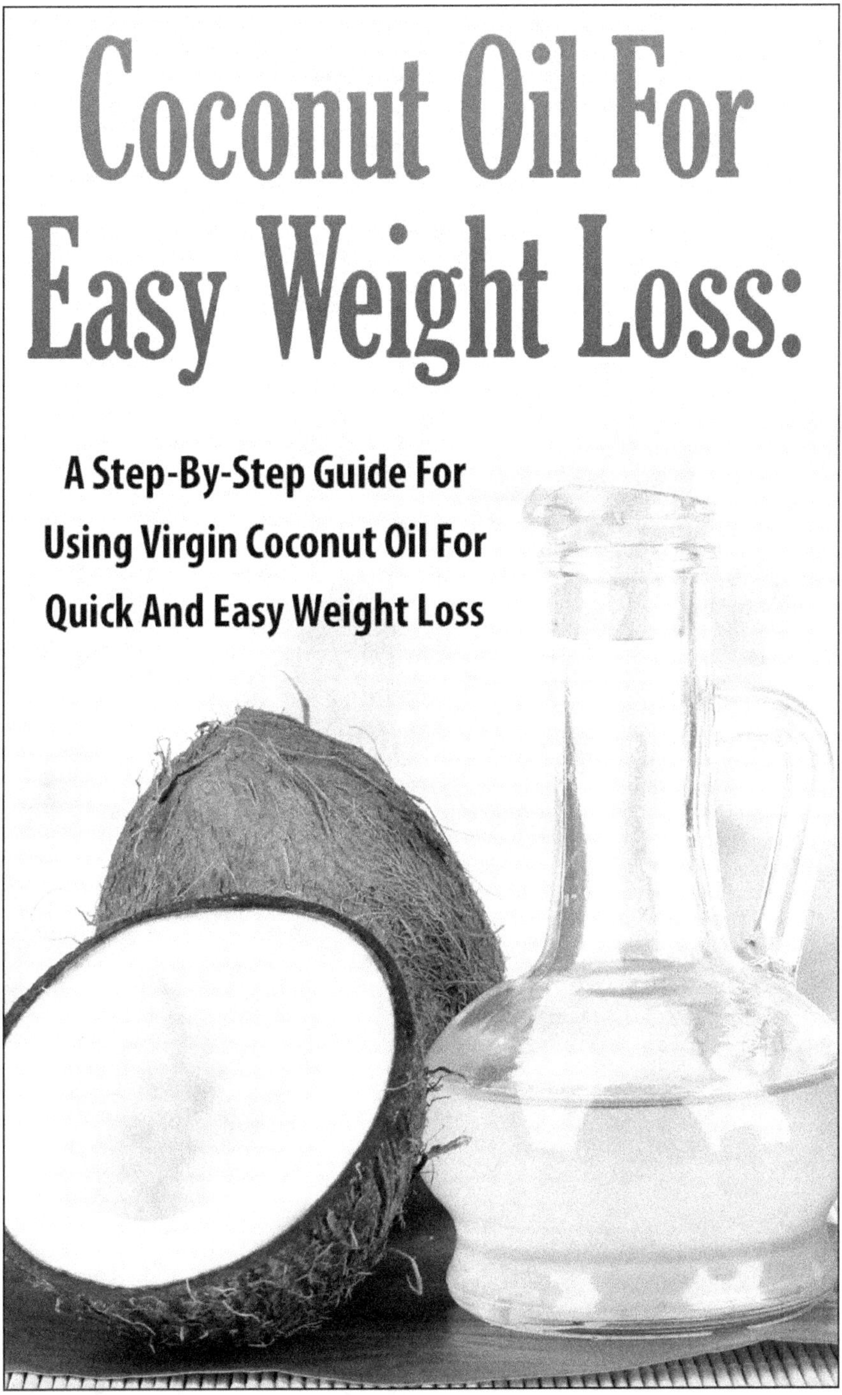

Coconut Oil For
Easy Weight Loss:

**A Step-By-Step Guide For
Using Virgin Coconut Oil For
Quick And Easy Weight Loss**

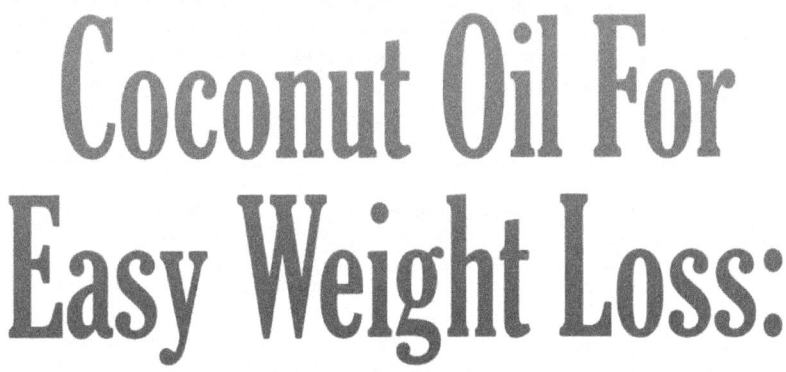

Table Of Contents

Introduction

I want to thank you and congratulate you for purchasing the ebook, *"Coconut Oil For Easy Weight Loss: A Step-By-Step Guide For Using Virgin Coconut Oil For Quick And Easy Weight Loss"*.

This book contains information on how Virgin Coconut Oil benefits our bodies as well as the different means through which it can hasten our weight loss. It is quite unconventional, considering that oil typically equals fat when we think about it. However, this is certainly not the case with coconut oil for it contains many beneficial nutrients that are good for our bodies—inside and out.

Here, you'll be provided with more than just simple facts. You'll also be given a few recipes that you can enjoy during your diet without having to worry that you'll end up ruining your routine. In fact, by eating these, you'll lose weight more efficiently.

Thanks again for purchasing this book. I hope you enjoy it!

Chapter 1: What is Virgin Coconut Oil?

Conventional thought used to consider different fats such as coconut oil to be just as unhealthy as animal fat and that consuming it would eventually lead to heart disease. However, we have since discovered that this is not true at all, and that coconut oil is actually very healthy for our cardiac system. It is quite unique, right? So what sets it apart from other oils? From food products such as butter and lard, which are also used for cooking but carries with it major health risks.

So what's in a coconut?

Coconuts, despite their humble appearance are actually excellent sources of nutrition. It can also be considered as a complete food with its healthy meal, oil and juice. Did you know that there are people who survive on nothing but the coconut? That's how great this often overlooked fruit is. Arguably, it's the oil that is the most nutritious and beneficial part of the fruit. With over 90% saturated fat content along with antifungal, antimicrobial and antibacterial properties, it's no wonder people use it from the inside to the outside.

How does Virgin Coconut Oil differ from other types of coconut oils?

What you must first know is that most commercial grade coconut oils are actually derived from copra or dried coconut meat. This can be made through various means such as sun drying, kiln drying as well as smoke drying. If dried coconut meat is used for the base material, the unrefined oil from it would not be fit for human consumption, at least not after it has been purified—or refined. This is because dried coconut meat can be very unsanitary considering the process through which it is made. The standard product derived from copra is called RBD coconut oil. RBD stands for refined, bleached and deodorized. There are chemicals used to make it.

On the other hand, virgin coconut oil is derived from fresh coconut meat; hence, it retains the scent and taste of the actual coconut. In fact, this is one of the ways through which you'd be able to differentiate it from an RBD. Because of the fact that it hasn't been processed and was derived through a sanitary manner, virgin coconut oil is considered to be much healthier and safer when it comes to human consumption. It must also be noted that it also retains far more of the good, healthy stuff that has made coconut oil a popular functional food by the medical community as well as health-conscious people all over the world.

More recently, however, it's being recognized for its effectiveness when it comes to hastening weight loss in people as well as lowering risks of heart disease development.

Medium Chain Fatty Acids (MCFA's)

A great majority of the fats that we consume are actually long chain fatty acids that the body needs to break down before we're able to absorb the nutrients we need from it. This takes a lot of work. On the other hand, the coconut oil contains high amounts of short and medium chain fatty acids which can be directly digested and sent to the liver in order to produce more energy for the body's use.

If you have diabetes, this is good for you as well. Because the MCFAs are sent directly to the liver, there is no need for our bodies to produce pancreatic enzymes or bile in order to digest it. This is one of the reasons why many experts recommend it for diabetics.

As for easy and efficient weight loss, the MCFA's serve a purpose as well.

MCFA's can, in fact, boost our metabolism along with our energy. So if you're exercising, this would provide you with a great advantage as you won't get tired easily. You'll also be able to quickly burn the food you eat and turn that into energy as well, enough to get you through the day or the exercise routines you intend to do.

What About Saturated Fat? Isn't that unhealthy?

Still concerned about this? While it does have quite the bad rep, it is worth considering that not all saturated fats are actually bad for the body. This is because they don't behave in the same way once we've consumed it. Take coconut oil for example. Because of its high Lauric acid content, it actually does more good than bad for us. This is apparent in the diets of many Thai people. They consume large amounts of saturated fats such as coconut oil and yet, they also have the lowest average when it comes to heart risk when compared to other countries.

Chapter 2: How Virgin Coconut Oil Works For Weight Loss

There are many negative connotations when it comes to coconut oil and it's very generous saturated fat content, but fortunately all of those old beliefs have been debunked. These days, people no longer avoid consuming and using coconut oil because they are more aware of its health benefits and among those—weight loss.

The trick is simple: Coconut oil helps in boosting our metabolism thus allowing our bodies to burn fat quicker and more efficiently.

With all the different dangers that are typically associated with thermogenic stimulants, it's not surprising that a lot of people tend to simply stay away from them. For weight watchers, this is an unfortunate thing because it does help them improve their metabolic rate as well as hasten the process itself. Luckily, they now have another alternative. Something more natural that wouldn't have them resorting to weight loss pills or overdosing on caffeine just to get the same effect. Extra virgin coconut oil is one of the safest options when it comes to losing weight quickly.

Earlier, we learned that coconut oil primarily consists of short and medium chain fatty acids and these are known to help in speeding up our metabolic rate. They are easily digestible and could be turned to energy without much trouble. In fact, a study was done in order to determine the act effects of these MCFA's on our metabolism. During the tests they conducted, where every participant's metabolic rate was evaluated, they were able to find out that coconut oil was able to increase the metabolism by at least 65%. The study also showed that contrary to what some people believe, the effects lasted for 24 hours max. This is a significant find, considering, the biggest disadvantage that many weight watchers have is a slow metabolism brought on by years of eating unhealthy food. If they are able to change that, well, the process itself should be much easier and quicker to accomplish.

There are other ways through which coconut oil can help when it comes to weight loss and maintaining a healthy weight. Below are a few examples:

1. Coconut oil helps in slowing down the digestion of our food and this can help us feel much fuller after a meal. If you add coconut oil to your diet, you can also help reduce the need to snack in between meals because you won't feel hungry easily. This helps you avoid overeating as well.

2. Because of its ability to help slow down the process of digestion, coconut oil can also help in preventing blood sugar fluctuations that tend to happen after we've eaten a rather heavy meal. So if you have a tendency to feel sleepy after lunch, consuming coconut oil together with your meal would allow you to avoid that.

3. The medium chain fatty acids found in coconut oil is also capable of destroying candida which is a condition wherein there's yeast overgrowth in the body. This would actually trigger weight gain as well as a craving for carbohydrates as well as induce fatigue. If you want to lose weight successfully, you need to eliminate this first. Only then will you be able to maintain your desired weight.

4. For detoxifying the body, coconut oil is also a great product to use. It helps in ridding the body of many infirmities as well as in balancing our digestive tract all while nourishing the healthy cells in our bodies. This simple process can help in restoring our body to its previous health while paving the way for a quick and easy weight loss.

Produces Energy and Not Fat

Whenever people go on diets as a means of losing weight, they would typically restrain themselves from eating foods which are known to contain the most amount of fat. But why is it singled out? Other than the fact that it increases the calories in our body, it is because of the way it is digested and used that contributes to the most amount of fat storage. Simply put, the fat we eat is also the fat that ends up on the thicker parts of our bodies.

Whenever we eat fat, it is broken down by the body into individual fatty acids and then bundled up into fat and protein called lipoproteins. These are then sent into our bloodstream where the fatty acids are directly deposited into our fat cells. Other nutrients such as protein and carbohydrate are also broken down but unlike the fatty acids, they are immediately utilized for energy or the building of body tissue. Only when we eat in excess of those two does it become converted into body fat.

MCFA's found in virgin coconut oil are digested and utilized differently, however. Unlike typical food fat, they are not bundled into lipoproteins or circulated in the bloodstream before ending up in storage (in your arms, thighs and tummy). Rather, they are actually converted into energy immediately much like the protein and carbs that you consume. So when you

101

consume virgin coconut oil, you gain more energy without having to worry about the fat getting stored in your body. This has been a well-documented fat that's been observed in both animals and humans. The research clearly shows that by replacing your usual oil with the virgin coconut variety, you will be able to decrease your body weight as well as reduce the amount of stored fat in your body.

Chapter 3: Other Known Health Benefits

Besides aiding in speedy weight loss, virgin coconut oil has a number of other health benefits. Among them are the following:

1. Alzheimer's and Other Neurological Diseases – The MCT's or medium chain triglycerides commonly found in virgin coconut oil are known to be helpful when it comes to improving our brain function.

2. Anti-aging – It is more effective than chemical-laden creams and lotions when it comes to smoothing out wrinkles, restoring the elasticity of saggy skin as well as decreasing the appearance of different age spots. It also works as a protective oxidant, warding off free radicals that are often the cause of premature aging as well as other degenerative skin diseases. Unlike other oils, it helps maintain the body's natural antioxidant reserves as well as protects our skin from harmful ultraviolet rays which can further increase wrinkle formation.

3. Improves Athletic Performance – It can serve as source of quick energy during training. At the same time, it helps improve an athlete's endurance as well as keep their energy levels up through natural means.

4. Bones – It aids the body in the absorption of different nutrients such as magnesium and calcium, both of which are needed by the body to develop strong bones as well as prevent osteoporosis.

5. Diabetes – Virgin coconut oil can help when it comes to controlling blood sugar levels as well as in improving the

body's ability to produce insulin. It can also help prevent and treat diabetes by enabling the body to utilize the blood glucose more efficiently. It can also provide ketones as an alternative source of energy and at the same time, effectively reduces the symptoms of diabetes along with lowering a person's risks of developing it.

6. Digestion – Improves the functions of our digestive system and helps prevent various stomach related problems which also includes IBS. It contains antimicrobial properties which can effectively fight off fungi, bacteria and parasites. All of which can cause serious indigestion. When it comes to mineral and nutrient absorption, it also makes the body more efficient and capable of taking the important stuff from the food that we eat. These also help if you're on a diet and trying to lose weight.

7. Hair Care – If used regularly on the hair, virgin coconut oil helps in making it grow healthier and shinier. It can also help in controlling dandruff as well as lice and lice eggs. If your hair has been significantly damaged by various treatments and you want it to go back to a much healthier state, regular application would hasten the regrowth and get rid of damaged parts. Along with that, it can also greatly nourish your hair with the nutrients it needs, thus making for a great all natural conditioner.

8. Heart Health – If you're worried about its effects on your heart then fret not because it actually contains "good fat" that will not accumulate in your arteries and clog them up. It will not raise your LDL unlike other vegetable oils would. In fact, it is comprised of 50% lauric acid which can actually help in lowering high blood pressure as well

as high cholesterol levels. In some cases, it has even reduced the risk of heart disease in people as well as prevented atherosclerosis.

9. Immune System – Virgin coconut oil contains lauric acid, antimicrobial lipids, caprylic acid as well as capric acid. These also have antibacterial, antifungal and antiviral properties that help in strengthening our immune systems. By taking it, you can also lower your risk of getting viral and bacterial infection, avoid influenza as well as be a bit more immune to cytomegalovirus and HIV. It also helps in treating and fighting off fungi and yeast which can cause ringworm problems, candidiasis, thrush, diaper rash and athlete's foot.

10. Kidney and Liver – When it comes to the kidney, not only will it aid in dissolving kidney stones, it can also help you prevent any related diseases. As for the liver, because of the MCFTA's contained in the virgin coconut oil, the liver needs to work less into converting it into energy therefore there isn't much strain on the organ itself.

11. Skin Care – Virgin coconut oil has a plethora of benefits when it comes to skin care. The first of which would be its ability to aid in the natural pH balance of the skin and helps in relieving any dryness or flaking brought on by an imbalance or dry weather. If you have oily skin, it is likely that you have a hard time looking for the right moisturizer for your skin. Look no further because coconut oil has the right elements for this purpose. It won't leave your skin feeling greasy. Besides those, it can

also help in reducing the symptoms of eczema, psoriasis, dermatitis as well as a number of other skin problems.

Chapter 4: Virgin Coconut Oil Diet Recipes

Alright, now that you know all about the different benefits that you can get from adding virgin coconut oil to your diet, you must be wondering about how you can do just that. If you're not too keen on taking the product directly, here are a few delicious ways through which you can add it to your daily menu.

Refreshing Smoothie Recipes:

I.   Berry Coconut Smoothie

This smoothie is significantly high in antioxidant amounts and is one of the best when it comes to mixing with coconut oil. The flavors work very well together to create a refreshing and sweet taste. Because of the high antioxidant content, it is recommended that you have it as a dessert after a meal or before bed. It will efficiently cleanse your body.

Ingredients: 1 tablespoon of raw virgin coconut oil. 1 cup of unsweetened almond milk or one that's vanilla flavored. A cup of strawberries, you can also mix it with other varieties such as blueberries or raspberries. 5 ice cubes. You can also add in a scoop of your favorite protein shake if you intend to turn it into a meal smoothie.

To make: Simply blend together and serve chilled.

II.   Island Dream Smoothie

This smoothie features spirulina, a protein-rich superfood. It has a rich, brilliant green color and by adding some stevia into it, a refreshing sweetness that also masks the earthy taste brought by the spirulina. If you're on a diet and still looking for something healthy to eat, this would be the best option to try. It contains many of the nutrients that your body needs for the day without the added calories!

Ingredients: A cup of coconut water (or a regular one, it depends on what you like). 1 to 2 tablespoons of raw virgin coconut oil depending on what you need. A tablespoon of organic spirulina powder mixed with half a cup of frozen banana and pineapples. A packet of NuNaturals Stevia or another brand that you prefer. A handful of spinach and at least 5 ice cubes.

To make: Simply blend and serve chilled.

III.   Superfood Smoothie

On the subject of superfoods, here's one that many weight watchers would certainly enjoy. This smoothie recipe contains 5 different superfoods that are needed on a daily basis when it comes to energy, hormonal balance, skin and metabolism. They are also significantly high when it comes to raw amino acids and would make for a great meal replacement, as a snack or even as an afternoon pick me up. It would make you feel full and energized but without the added calories and fats!

Ingredients: A cup of unsweetened vanilla coconut milk or almond milk depending on your tastes. ¼ cup of frozen blueberries. A teaspoon of maca powder and raw cacao powder as well as a teaspoon of your favorite green powder, doesn't matter which brand. 1 scoop of protein powder, use your favorite! 1 teaspoon of acai powder or goji powder if that's something you like more. 1 teaspoon of vanilla extract, make sure it's gluten free. 2 tablespoons of virgin coconut oil and add a handful of spinach. Lastly, 5 to 6 pieces ice cubes.

To make: Blend, chill and serve.

IV.   Coconut Acai Smoothie

Acai, another well-known superfood makes an appearance in this delicious and very filling smoothie. It contains a lot of Omega 3 fatty acids, protein as well as a generous amount of antioxidants which is great for speeding up your metabolism and of course, hastening weight loss as well. If you air that with the different health benefits that virgin coconut oil can offer and you've got yourself a smoothie that could easily replace a meal. Have it as a snack or drink it for breakfast!

Ingredients: 1 cup of unsweetened coconut milk or almond milk. 1 frozen packet of acai pulp as well as 2 tablespoons of coconut oil. 1 packet of Stevia powder as well as a dash or vanilla or cinnamon for added sweetness and flavor.

To make: Simply blend and serve.

V.   Coconut and Kale Smoothie

Kale and coconut may seem like an unlikely pair but they do make for a refreshing and filling green smoothie that could easily replace any of your meals for the day. It contains proteins as well as different vitamins, iron and fiber as well as Omega 3's. All of which are enough to power you through the day. You can have it from breakfast or as a dessert after one of your meals. It would make you feel as if you've just snacked on a really delicious salad.

Ingredients: 1 cup of unsweetened vanilla milk or coconut milk if this is more of your taste. You will also need 1 cup of kale, 1 cup of spinach as well as half a frozen banana. ¼ cup of frozen blueberries, 1 to 2 tablespoons of virgin coconut oil along with a dash of cinnamon. Lastly, add 5 ice cubes into the mix.

To make: Simply blend and chill before serving.

Meals and Desserts:

I. Coconut Fried Shrimp

If you're looking to change up your meals to something much healthier and more appropriate when it comes to weight loss then this recipe is something you should try. Filling, delicious and low in calories, you're sure to enjoy it.

Ingredients: You will need a pound of peeled fresh shrimp. ½ cup of organic coconut flour. ¼ cup of organic cornstarch mixed with ½ a teaspoon of fine salt. You will also need ½ a cup of water, 2 eggs and ½ cups of organic shredded coconut. Add ½ cup of virgin coconut oil and ½ cup of virgin palm oil to the mix and you're done.

To make: Mix the starch, the coconut flour, salt, water and the eggs in a bowl. Using a fork, blend it all together until the starches get dissolved. Dip the shrimp in this simple batter before rolling it onto the shredded coconut. Heat your palm and coconut oils in a skillet at about 375 degrees then fry the shrimp until it becomes golden brown. A minute for each side should be enough because if you overcook shrimp, it can easily become a little rubbery in texture. To remove the excess oil, simply drain the shrimp on paper towels before you serve it. As an alternative to the palm oil, you can also make use of organic palm shortening instead.

II. Coconut Chicken Strips with Honey Mustard

Typically, fried chicken isn't something dieters would want to touch but with this recipe, you'll be able to enjoy this delicious food guilt free while getting to enjoy the benefits of consuming coconut oil as well. Here's what you need to do:

Ingredients: 1 ½ cups of coconut chips or shredded coconut depending on your preferences. 1 ½ pounds of organic chicken breasts that has been cut into strips, this is the healthiest part of the chicken. You will also need 2 tablespoons of butter, olive and virgin coconut oil. 1 tablespoon of flour mixed with 1 teaspoon of nutmeg. Lastly, you'll need ½ a cup of prepared mustard and 2 tablespoons of honey.

To make: To get started, turn your own on and set it to broil. Set your coconut shreds evenly on a baking sheet and toast this until it becomes slightly browned. Removed from the oven and let it cool to one side. Next, pre-heat your own to 375 degrees and while that's heating up, mix your flour, nutmeg and the toasted coconut into one bowl. Place your chicken strips in there and drizzle it with the coconut oil. You can skip using butter for this recipe if you don't like it. Prepare your cookie sheet by putting some of the coconut oil on it as well; this is so it doesn't end up sticking while it cooks. Coat your chicken evenly with the dry mixture before you bake it. Leave it baking for at least ten minutes or until it becomes thoroughly cooked. After, prepare the mustard and honey by simply mixing both together.

III.   Peanut Butter Granola With Coconut Oil

If you're looking for something sweet yet healthy to satisfy your sweet tooth then this recipe would surely whet your appetite.

Ingredients: 1/3 cup of raw honey as well as ½ cup of peanut butter. You will also need a tablespoon of coconut cream and ¼ cup of coconut oil. Add 2 cups of oatmeal to that along with ¾ cup of coconut flakes.

To make: Making this dessert snack is actually pretty simple and would take very little time. To get started, preheat your oven to 275 degrees. Then, mix all of your ingredients together, except for the coconut and oatmeal, in a saucepan. Make sure that you keep it at a very low heat. Mix this until it becomes smooth. Once the consistency is to your liking, simply add the oatmeal and coconut flakes. Stir these in well. Spread the mixture onto an oiled cookie sheet and put it in the preheated oven for at least 10 minutes. Stir it once more and get the air bubbles to pop before putting it back in for another 10 minutes. Once done, let it cool before serving. This recipe is best eaten with milk and would be great snacks between your meals whenever you're craving.

IV.   Gluten-free Zucchini Pancakes

Looking for a refreshing lunch or something to snack on in-between your meals? This recipe would certainly fit great into that need.

Ingredients: 1 medium stalk zucchini, make sure that the ends have been removed and have it coarsely grated. You will also need 2 eggs, 2 to 3 tablespoons of virgin coconut oil as well as a teaspoon of red onion that's been finely chopped. Freshly ground black pepper, 2 teaspoons of asiago cheese that's been grated, this would add flavor to the meal. 2 to 3 basil leaves, finely minced. Lastly, you will also need a teaspoon of coconut flour and a dash of salt to taste.

To make: In a bowl, add your grated zucchini and eggs together, mix it thoroughly and make sure everything is coated. Heat your coconut oil in a large skillet then add black pepper, onion, asiago cheese, and some basil to your zucchini. If the mixture is a little too liquid for your liking, add a few dashes of the coconut oil to thicken it. When the oil is hot enough, carefully fork some of the batter into the pan and then mash it down to spread it. Make sure that you do this evenly so you make pancakes that aren't too thin. Let each side cook for about a minute or two, or up until it becomes a deeper brown shade. Once completely cooked, drain the excess oil on paper towels before serving.

Chapter 5: Complement Your Virgin Coconut Oil Regimen

So there you have it, a step by step guide to learning more about virgin coconut oil and its many different uses, including how it can help you lose weight. Remember, it's important to learn the basics before you get started as there is a difference between regular coconut oil and the virgin variety. As you have learned, the latter is healthier and supports many of the health benefits that your body needs, especially if you're trying to lose weight and changing up your diet.

Keep these in mind:

To lose weight using virgin coconut oil, it doesn't necessarily mean that you simply have to consume it and wait for the results. It would still require a bit of work.

1. Change your diet into something healthier and incorporate virgin coconut oil into your daily menu using some of the recipes provided above. Be disciplined, however, and avoid overindulging. But because coconut oil would help you feel fuller for longer, snacking can be easily avoided.

2. Do exercise. Simply eating virgin coconut oil is not enough to do the trick. Add a regular exercise routine to your everyday tasks. It doesn't have to be tedious but you will need to sweat and use your muscles for it. Brisk walking, yoga, or something as simple as going up and down the first two steps of the stairs would be good enough as long as you do it every day.

3. Lastly, make the necessary lifestyle changes. There are certain habits that we have which can hinder weight loss. Look at your habits, cross out the bad ones and simply change them into something better.

Conclusion

Thank you again for purchasing this book!

I hope this book was able to help you to better understand how virgin coconut oil benefits our health and body, as well as how it can help dieters achieve their weight loss goals without compromising their good health.

The next step is to apply all that you have learned in this eBook and watch the transformation happen on you.

Finally, if you enjoyed this book, please take the time to share your thoughts and post a review on Amazon. We do our best to reach out to readers and provide the best value we can. Your positive review will help us achieve that. It'd be greatly appreciated!

Thank you and good luck!

Book 5:

Homemade Body Scrubs & Masks for Beginners

BY LINDSEY P

50 Proven All Natural, Easy Recipes for Body Scrub & Facial Masks to Exfoliate, Nourish, & Care for Your Skin

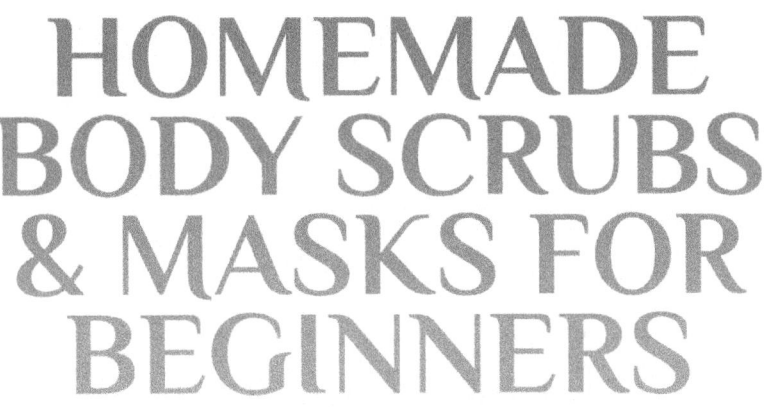

HOMEMADE BODY SCRUBS & MASKS FOR BEGINNERS

50 Proven All Natural, Easy Recipes For Body Scrubs & Facial Masks To exfoliate, Nourish & Care For You Skin

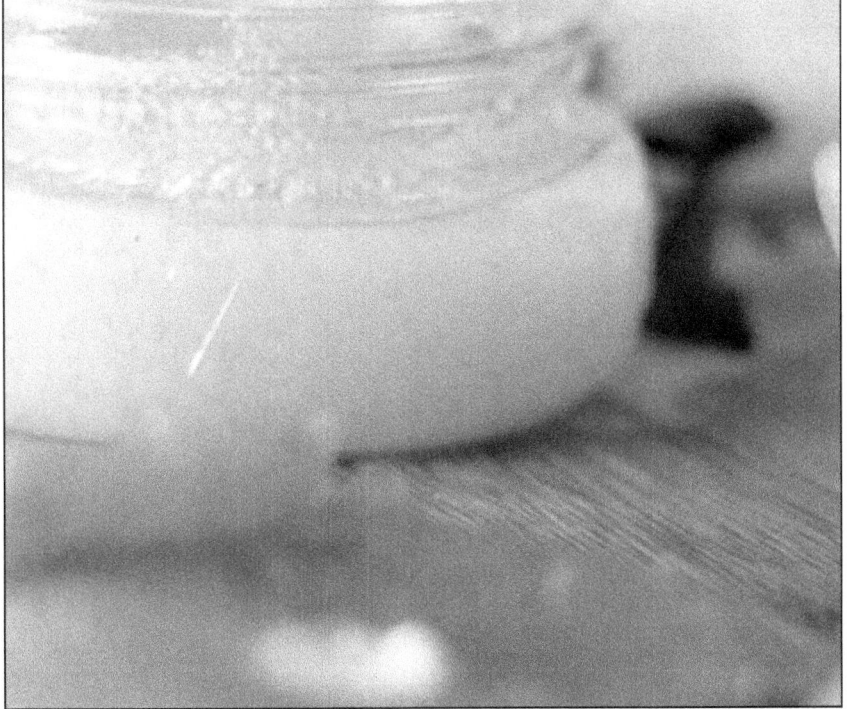

Table Of Contents

Introduction

I want to thank you and congratulate you for purchasing the book, *"Homemade Bodyscrubs & Masks for Beginners: 50 Proven all Natural, Easy Recipes for Body Scrubs & Facial Masks to Exfoliate, Nourish, & Care for Your Skin"*.

This book contains proven steps and strategies on how to create effective body scrubs and facial masks using a multitude of organic and natural products.

Exfoliation should always be a part of your skincare routine. This helps unclog your pores, slough off dull skin, balance sebum production, and even out your complexion. Importantly, exfoliation keeps the skin healthy, young-looking, and more glowing.

The good news is that you don't have to purchase expensive exfoliants and masks to have beautiful skin. You can easily make your own scrubs with the use different items that are found in your home and garden. By creating your own skincare product, you can be sure that the ingredients are not just effective but safe and natural too. Try makes these body scrubs and facial masks today!

Thanks again for purchasing this book, I hope you enjoy it!

Chapter 1: Sugar Body Scrubs

Banana & Sugar Scrub

Ingredients: 1 very ripe banana, ¼ teaspoon vanilla extract (pure), and 3 tablespoons granulated sugar

Directions: Combine all the ingredients together in a bowl. Mash the banana chunkily. Apply all over the body in a gentle, massaging motion. Rinse after 10-15 minutes.

Main ingredient: Banana

Bananas high Vitamin B6 and C content maintains and improves the elasticity of the skin. Its anti-oxidants also protect the skin from free radical damage and premature aging. It also helps hydrate the skin to make it suppler and prevent peeling.

Coconut Vanilla Sugar Scrub

Ingredients: ½ teaspoon fresh vanilla, ½ cup coconut oil, and ½ cup brown sugar

Mix all the ingredients together in a bowl or jar. Massage on your entire body for a few minutes before rinsing. You may also use the scrub as a massage cream.

Main Ingredient: coconut oil

Coconut oil is very effective in moisturizing and softening skin. Its antibacterial properties ward off bacteria and hasten healing. The antioxidants found in coconut oil also reduces appearance of wrinkles, thwart cellular aging.

Peppermint Coco Scrub

Ingredients: ½ cup coconut oil, 1 cup sugar, 1 tablespoon powdered milk, 2 drops peppermint essential oil, and 2-3 drops green food coloring (optional)

Directions: Combine all the ingredients, except the oil, in a container. Mix well. Add in the peppermint essential oil and stir thoroughly. Massage into the skin for a few minutes. Rinse with warm water.

Main ingredients: coconut oil and peppermint essential oil

Coconut oil helps moisturize and hydrate the skin to keep it supple and young- looking. Peppermint essential oil is cool and very refreshing. It revitalizes dull skin and removes excess oil to keeps back acne at bay.

Lavender Vanilla Scrub

Ingredients: ½ cup melted coconut oil, 4 tablespoons sweet almond oil, 15 drops lavender essential oil, 1 teaspoon fresh vanilla, and 1 cup white sugar

Directions: Transfer the sugar into a bowl. Mix in the sweet almond oil and coconut oil. Next, stir in the lavender essential oil and vanilla. Massage the scrub all over the body. Leave on for 20 to 30 minutes before rinsing with warm water.

Main ingredient: lavender essential oil

Lavender essential oil's scent effectively soothes and calms the mind and body. This essential oil also has antiseptic properties that heals acne and wounds, minimizes redness and swelling, and reduces appearance of scars. It also increases blood

circulation, firms the skin, and relieves sore muscles and cramps.

Cinna-Choco Scrub

Ingredients: ½ cup white sugar, 1 cup brown sugar, ½ tablespoon cocoa powder, ½ tablespoon cinnamon powder, and 2 tablespoons olive oil.

Directions: Combine all the ingredients in a bowl and stir well. Apply on the skin and massage in a circular motion. Rinse with warm water.

Main ingredient: cocoa powder

Cocoa powder is full of anti-oxidants that help protect the skin from free radical damage. Its natural exfoliants also remove dead skin cells to achieve a more glowing complexion.

Citrusy Fresh Scrub

Ingredients: 20 drops lime essential oil, 3 drops orange essential oil, 5 drops lemon essential oil, 3 drops bergamot essential oil, 1/3 cup melted virgin coconut oil, ½ cup carrier oil (jojoba oil or safflower oil), and 2 cups sugar

Directions: Except for the carrier oil, stir all the ingredients in the bowl. Slowly add the carrier oil into the mixture until you've reached the appropriate consistency. Massage unto the skin and rinse thoroughly.

Main ingredient: lemon and lime essential oils

Lemon and lime essential oils both have astringent, anti-bacterial, and antiseptic properties. It is quite effective in reducing sebum production and preventing and treating acne.

These essential oils also have anti-aging properties to reduce appearance of wrinkles and maintain a youthful glow.

Sugar Coffee Scrub

Ingredients: ¼ cup ground coffee, ¼ cup raw brown sugar, 2 tablespoons virgin coconut oil, 1 tablespoon olive oil, and 1 tablespoon sea salt

Directions: Combine all the ingredients thoroughly. Grab a handful of the scrub and massage your body in a circular motion for several minutes. Rinse with warm water.

Main ingredient: ground coffee

Ground coffee effectively reduces the appearance of cellulite. This is because the antioxidants and caffeine in the coffee increases blood circulation in the body and dilates the blood vessels. The grounds also exfoliate the skin to make it luminous and supple.

Coco Ginger Scrub

Ingredients: 1 tablespoon coarsely chopped peeled ginger root, ¼ cup sunflower oil, ¼ cup coconut oil, ¼ cup kosher salt, ¾ cup granulated sugar, and 4 drops lemongrass essential oil

Directions: Using a small pan, heat ginger and coconut oil over a low flame for 10 minutes. This will allow the oils and scent of the ginger to mix with the oil. Turn off the heat and filter the liquid into a bowl. Discard the ginger bits.

Mix in the sunflower oil into the warm ginger-infused oil. Stir well and add the salt and sugar. Stir and add the lemongrass essential oil. Massage this scrub all over the body and leave on for 5 minutes. Rinse as usual.

Main ingredient: ginger root

A favorite home remedy, ginger root possesses anti-inflammatory properties that help heal a variety of skin diseases, prevent acne, reduce swelling, and stop redness. Its antioxidant properties also make the skin tight, glowing, and energized.

Easy Vanilla Sugar Scrub

Ingredients: ¼ cup white sugar, ½ cup brown sugar, ¼ cup sweet almond oil, and 3 tablespoons vanilla extract

Directions: Combine the brown and white sugars in a mixing bowl. Add the sweet almond oil and vanilla extract. Stir well. Apply the body scrub on damp skin and massage for several minutes until the sugars dissolve. Rinse with warm water.

Main ingredient: vanilla extract

Not just used for baked goods, vanilla is chockfull of antioxidants, vitamins and minerals. It improves your skin tone, hastens wound healing, soothes irritated skin, and prevents premature aging.

Spice-y Scrub

Ingredients: ¾ cup almond oil, 2 teaspoons ginger powder, 2 teaspoons cinnamon powder, 2 teaspoons nutmeg powder, 1 cup granulated sugar, and 1 cup brown sugar

Directions: Put all the dry ingredients first in a bowl. Add the oil and whisk together thoroughly. Massage into the skin and rinse after a several minutes.

Main ingredients: ginger, cinnamon, and nutmeg

Ginger naturally prevents premature skin aging, reduces appearance of wrinkles and sagging skin, fights infections, calms swelling, and purifies and smoothens the skin. Cinnamon contains antimicrobial and antiseptic properties that aid in fighting infections and warding off bad odor. Nutmeg helps reduce blackheads and makes scars lighter and less noticeable. It also offers relief from muscle and joint pain.

Reviving Vanilla Scrub

Ingredients: juice of 3 lemon, 15 vanilla beans, 9 drops vanilla essential oil, and 9 tablespoons brown sugar.

Directions: Get your vanilla beans and slice them lengthwise to open. Use a spoon to scrape out the seeds and transfer to a mixing bowl. Add in the lemon juice and stir. Mix in the brown sugar and essential oil. Stir well. Apply the scrub on the body and massage well. Rinse with warm water and follow with cold water.

Main ingredient: vanilla essential oil

Vanilla is always a favorite when it comes to soothing scents but its benefits go beyond its fragrance. Vanilla contains anti-inflammatory components that stop and soothe swelling. Its antibacterial properties kill acne and body odor causing bacteria, boost wound healing, and reduce infections.

Vitamin Lavender Scrub

Ingredients: 1 tablespoon Vitamin E, 3 tablespoons almond oil, ½ cup coconut oil (organic), and 1/3 cup Celtic sea salt, 1 cup cane sugar (organic), and lavender essential oil

Directions: Combine the salt and sugar in a bowl. Add in the coconut oil and almond oil. Mix well. Stir in the vitamin E and the 9 drops of lavender essential oil. Scrub on wet skin and rinse with warm water after a few minutes.

Main ingredients: lavender and vitamin E

Lavender is widely used for its calming and cleansing properties. It helps stop itching and swelling caused by insect bites and stings, minor burns, and minor wound bleeding. Vitamin E is a powerful antioxidant that stops premature skin aging and further cell damage. It promotes younger looking skin that's supple and healthy.

Milk Body Scrub

Ingredients: 2 tablespoons fresh whole milk, 2 tablespoons light vegetable oil, ½ cup granulated white sugar

Directions: Combine all the ingredients in a bowl. Mix well until creamy. Rub on damp skin and leave on for 25-30 minutes. Rinse with warm water.

Main ingredient: milk

Milk improves skin complexion by making it fairer, brighter, and softer. It also cleanses the skin while reducing the size of the pores. Milk naturally restores the skin's moisture to keep it supple and young-looking.

Spicy Sugar Scrub

Ingredients: ¾ cup sugar, 2 tablespoons fresh orange zest, 2 tablespoons ground cloves, 1 tablespoon dried rose petals, and 1 ½ cups sesame oil

Directions: Using a bowl, mix all the ingredients thoroughly. Apply on damp skin and massage for several minutes. Rinse well.

Main ingredient: ground cloves

Ground cloves reduce inflammation symptoms and provide a mild anesthetic effect to subdue body and muscle pain.

Matcha Sugar Scrub

Ingredients: 1 teaspoon matcha green tea powder, 1 tablespoon green tea (from tea bags), 1 cup granulate sugar, ½ cup coconut oil

Directions: Combine all the ingredients together in a bowl. Massage on damp skin for several minutes before rinsing.

Main ingredient: green tea

Full of antioxidants, green tea firms and tones the skin to make it look younger. It fights redness and irritation from various skin diseases like rosacea, psoriasis or eczema.

Chapter 2: Salt Body Scrubs

Coarse Lavender Salt Scrub

Ingredients: 1/3 cup grapeseed oil, 1 tablespoon dried lavender,16 drops lavender essential oil, and ½ cup coarse sea salt

Directions: Put the sea salt in a mixing bowl and pour in the grapeseed oil. Stir the ingredients together. Mix in the dried lavender. Add the essential oil and combine well. Apply on wet skin and massage gently. Do not use this scrub if you have any open wounds or cuts.

Main ingredient: lavender

When used in aromatherapy, the scent of lavender eliminates stress and anxiety. If applied on the skin, it offers an analgesic and sedative effect that eliminates minor aches and pains. Lavender's astringent properties minimize swelling too.

Thyme Lemon Salt Scrub

Ingredient: 2 teaspoons fresh thyme leaves, zest of a whole lemon, ½ cup organic almond oil, and 1 cup plain kosher salt

Directions: Pour the salt in a bowl. Add in the thyme leaves and lemon zest. Mix in the almond oil. Combine all ingredients thoroughly. Massage on damp skin and leave on for 20 minutes before rinsing with warm water.

Main ingredients: thyme and lemon

Thyme is very beneficial to the skin. It helps reduce

inflammation, heals lesions, and kills acne-causing bacteria. Lemon is also equally beneficial because it brightens the skin, reduces age spots, makes blackheads disappear, and stop excess oil production.

Tea Tree Salt Scrub

Ingredients: 3 teaspoons 15% tea tree oil and 1 cup kosher salt

Directions: Place a kosher salt in a bowl. Add in the tea tree oil and mix well. Apply on wet skin and massage gently. Leave on for several minutes and rinse. If using on dry skin, add a few drops of water to a handful of scrub and apply. Leave on until dry and brush off.

Main ingredient: tea tree oil

Tea tree oil contains anti-inflammatory properties that treat acne and inflamed skin allergies. Its anti-bacterial components can cure athlete's foot, skin dandruff, and other bacterial skin ailments.

Sage Salt Scrub

Ingredients: 4-7 fresh sage leaves, ½ cup date sugar, 1 cup olive oil, fresh zest of 1 grapefruit, and 2 cups fine sea salt

Directions: Place the sage and olive oil in the blender and process on high. Transfer the pureed mixture in a bowl and add the date sugar and sea salt. Stir well. Add the grapefruit zest and mix thoroughly. Apply the scrub on the skin and massage for two minutes. Rinse well.

Main ingredient: sage leaves

Sage leaves extract are often added to many skin care products because of their efficacy. Rich in vitamin A and calcium, it helps in daily cell regeneration to stop premature aging and wrinkles. It also improves blood circulation in the body to reduce varicose veins and cellulite. Sage also hastens healing of skin disorders including psoriasis and eczema symptoms.

Citrus Salt Scrub

Ingredients: 6 tablespoons iodized salt, 2 tablespoons Epsom salt, 2 cups white sugar, citrus essential oil (grapefruit, sweet orange, or lemon), and 1 cup jojoba oil

Directions: Put the salt and sugar inside the blender or food processor. Pulse several times to make the crystals finer. Transfer the mixture in a bowl. Add the jojoba oil and whisk to combine. Add about 25-30 drops of the citrus essential oil and mix. Use on this scrub on wet skin. Massage in circular motions and rinse well.

Main ingredient: Epsom salt and citrus essential oil

A popular natural remedy, Epsom salt contains magnesium and sulfate that reduces inflammation, improves muscle function, flushes out toxins, and increases nutrient absorption. Citrus essential oils are wide used for their light and refreshing aromas. Their scent uplifts the mood and energizes the body. When applied on the skin, it helps fight acne and prevent oily skin.

Scented Epsom Scrub

Ingredients: 1 cup Epsom salt, 1 cup sweet almond oil, and 10 drops rose essential oil

Directions: Combine all the ingredients in a small bowl. Mix well until a thick texture is achieved. Scrub all over your wet skin and massage gently. Rinse well and pat to dry.

Main ingredient: rose essential oil

Rose essential oil is commonly used in many skin care products because of its appealing scent. Apart from this, the oil also reduces appearance of stretch marks and scars, regenerates healthy skin cells, moisturizes very dry skin, and heals symptoms of eczema.

Salt Floral Scrub

Ingredients: 1 cup sea salt, 1 tablespoon dried rose, 7 drops rose hip seed oil, and ½ cup sweet almond oil

Directions: Mix the salt and oils in the bowl. Add in the dried rose and crush gently. Apply on the skin and massage for several minutes. Rinse well.

Main ingredient: dried rose

Dried rose contains beta carotene and B vitamins that help keeps skin fresh, moisturized, and healthy. It also reduces swelling and fights various skin infections.

Pumpkin Scrub

Ingredients: ½ cup pure pumpkin puree, 1 cup sea salt, 1 tablespoon sweet almond oil, and 1 teaspoon honey.

Directions: Mix the all the ingredients together. If you want the mixture to be oilier, add more almond oil.

Main ingredient: pumpkin puree

Perfect for all skin types, pumpkin contains a lot of vitamins that aid in healing, stopping free radical damage, and alleviating skin dryness. Its enzymes and anti-oxidants nourish the skin while removing dead skin cells.

Chapter 3: Salt and Sugar Free Body Scrubs

Oatmeal Chamomile Scrub

Ingredients: 4 tablespoons ground almonds, 1 tablespoon cornstarch, 4 tablespoons oatmeal, 1 tablespoon chamomile flowers, 2 tablespoons sweet almond oil, and 5 drops lavender extract

Directions: Place the ground almonds, cornstarch and oatmeal in a spice grinder or blender. Add the chamomile flowers and process well. Mix in the sweet almond oil and lavender extract. Stir well. To use, get a handful of the scrub and add several drops of water. Massage on damp skin for several minutes and wash off with warm water.

Main ingredient: ground almonds and chamomile flowers

Almonds are rich in phytochemicals that treat pimples, acne, and other skin conditions. It also reduces sebum production and prevents overly oily skin. Chamomile's anti-inflammatory and antiseptic properties soothe skin redness and swelling brought upon by acne, eczema, and minor burns.

Firming Scrub

Ingredients: 2 egg whites, 2 bay leaves, 1 celery stalk, ½ cup unpeeled cucumber slices, ¼ cup wheat germ, ½ cup hearts of palm (chopped), ¼ cup full-fat powdered milk, ¼ unpeeled russet potato slices, 1 teaspoon mint leaves, 1 teaspoon coconut extract, and 1 teaspoon vanilla extract

Ingredients: Place all the ingredients in a blender. Process until all the contents takes on a thick consistency. Apply all over the

137

body and massage for several minutes. Leave on for 20 minutes before rinsing with lukewarm water.

Main ingredient: russet potato, and celery

Russet potatoes naturally brighten the skin's complexion, refresh tired skin, remove dark spots, and nourish very dry skin. It also prevent acne, heal insect stings and bites, and soothe minor burns. Celery contains powerful antioxidants that delay skin aging, protect from free radical damage, and hydrates from the inside out. It also maintains the skin luminosity and elasticity.

Honey Wheat Germ Scrub

Ingredients: 2 tablespoons clear honey, 1 tablespoon wheat germ, 1 teaspoon sunflower oil, and 1 teaspoon fresh lemon juice

Directions: In small bowl, combine the wheat germ and the honey. Add the sunflower oil and lemon juice to the mixture. Stir well. Scrub on damp skin for several minutes. Rinse thoroughly.

Main ingredient: wheat germ

Wheat germ is rich in zinc which helps in skin cell production. It also contains anti-inflammatory properties that stop symptoms of eczema and other skin diseases and lessen acne swelling.

Almond Meal Scrub

Ingredients: ½ cup ground almond meal,1/2 cup oats (finely ground oats), and rosewater

Directions: Place the oats and almonds in the blender. Process them until well-combined. Transfer into a small bowl. Gently pour in the rosewater drop by drop until a paste is formed. Apply on damp skin and massage for several minute. Leave on skin for 30 minutes before rinsing.

Main ingredient: almond meal

Almond meal helps smoothen and soften the skin and removes dead skin cells. It also reduces swelling and clarifies skin complexion.

Chapter 4: Facial Masks for All Skin Types

Natural Banana Mask

Ingredients: 1/2 very ripe banana, 1 teaspoon Vitamin E oil, and 1 tablespoon yogurt

Directions: Mash the banana in a bowl and mix in the Vitamin E and yogurt. Apply it on a clean face and leave on for 30 minutes. Rinse with lukewarm water.

Main Ingredient: Banana

The banana is natural skin moisturizer. Its Vitamin C, B6, and A content help keeps the skin elastic and hydrated while repairing any skin damage.

Moisturizing Orange Mask

Ingredients: juice from 1 orange, 2 teaspoons dried orange peel, ½ cup oatmeal (steel-cup type), 3 tablespoons plain Greek yogurt, and 2 tablespoons honey

Directions: Gather all the ingredients and pour them in a bowl. Stir until well-combined. The consistency should be thick not runny. Apply the mask on a clean face. Leave on for 30 minutes and rinse with warm water.

Main ingredient: Orange

Oranges, especially its peels, has high vitamin C content. This vitamin is very effective in keeping the skin healthy and eliminating blemishes and dark spots. The citric acid in the

acid helps remove excess dirt and oil on the skin. It also dries up acne faster and reduces appearance of pimple marks. The essential oils found in the orange peel also rejuvenate and brighten skin, improve skin color and texture, and improve sagging skin.

Honey Almond Mask

Ingredients: 1 tablespoon honey and 3 almonds

Directions: Soak the almonds in water overnight. Place the soaked almonds in the blender and grind them finely. Remove from blender and transfer to a clean bowl. Slowly add a spoonful of honey into the ground almonds and stir well. Add a few drops of water until a paste is formed. Apply on a clean face and massage on a circular motion. Leave on for 30 minutes before rinsing with warm water and then, cold water.

Main ingredient: almonds

Almonds are rich in vitamin E. It protects the skin from the sun's ultraviolet rays, nourishes the skin to keep it moisturized and supple, and slows down aging.

Peach Facial Mask

Ingredients: 1 egg white and 1 very ripe peach

Directions: Put the peach in a food processor and puree until thick. Whisk the egg white until stiff peaks form and gently fold in the pureed peach. Apply to the face and neck. Leave on for 20-25 minutes and rinse with warm water.

Main ingredient: peach

Peach does wonders for tired and dried skin. Its high Vitamin C and A contents keep the skin healthy and refreshed. It moisturizes dry skin, regenerates skin cells, and brightens the complexion.

Pore Tightener Mask

Ingredients: 1 egg, 1 tablespoon organic honey, 1 teaspoon finely chopped fresh mint leaves, and 1 teaspoon crushed dried chamomile flowers

Directions: In a small bowl, whisk the egg and honey together. Add the rest of the ingredients and stir well. Massage on clean skin and let dry. Wash off with warm water and then, a splash of cold water.

Main ingredients: chamomile and mint leaves

Chamomile flowers contain healing, cleansing, and moisturizing properties which make it a really effective skin care treatment. It soothes sunburn, eliminates acne scars, hastens healing of minor wounds, reduces dark eye circles, and stops premature aging. The mint leaves' astringent properties soothe itching and infected skin, strengthen the facial skin tissue, and reduces sebum production. It also cleanses the skin to prevent clogged pores and promote clearer skin.

Cocoa Coffee Rejuvenating Mask

Ingredients: 5 tablespoons cocoa powder, 5 tablespoons freshly ground coffee, 8 tablespoons Greek yogurt, and 2 tablespoons raw honey

Directions: Slightly warm the honey in a small bowl. Add in the rest of the ingredients and mix well. Apply on the face and let set for 15 minutes. Rinse well.

Main ingredient: Coffee

Coffee increases blood circulation on the skin to give a rosy, healthy glow. It also tightens the skin and fights premature skin aging. The smell also revitalizes the soul and senses.

Chapter 5: Facial Masks for Oily and Acne-Prone Skin

Citrus Yogurt Mask

Ingredients: 1 cup yogurt (plain, not non-fat), 1 teaspoon carrot juice, 1 teaspoon fresh orange juice, and 1 teaspoon fresh lemon juice

Directions: Combine all the ingredients in a bowl. Apply to clean face and leave on for 10 minutes. Wipe off with washcloth dipped in warm water. Follow up rinse with cold water.

Main ingredient: orange and lemon juice

Orange and lemon juice contains a lot of nutrients that keep the skin fresh and young-looking. It effectively protects again free radical damage too. Lemon juice also lightens skin and reduces appearance of acne scars. The acid in these citrus juices mildly cleanses and removes excess oil.

Strawberry Mask

Ingredients: 9 strawberries and 3 tablespoons honey

Directions: Place the strawberries in a bowl and roughly mash with a fork. Add the honey and combine well. Apply on the face and leave on for several minutes before rinsing.

Main ingredient: strawberries

Strawberries effectively cleanses the skin while tightening the pores and sloughing off dead skin cells. It also regulates oil production and reduces appearance of acne.

Plum Almond Mask

Ingredients: 5-6 plums and 1 teaspoon almond oil

Directions: Boil the plums in water until soft. Transfer to a bowl and mash. Add the almond oil and combine well. Massage on the face for several minutes and rinse when dry.

Main ingredient: plums

Full of vitamin E , plums effectively prevent wrinkles and loss of skin elasticity. It also lightens dark spots, freckles, and other skin discoloration.

Peppermint Mask

Ingredients: 2 teaspoon dried peppermint, 2 teaspoon dried lavender, ½ cup almonds, 1/2 cup rolled oats, and ½ cups white cosmetic clay

Directions: Place the oats, almonds, and dried herbs in the spice grinder or high powered food processor. Grind into a very fine powder. Transfer the ground mixture in a bowl and add in the cosmetic clay. Mix well. Get a handful of the mixture and slowly add several drops of water to turn it into paste. Apply on the skin and leave on for 10 to 15 minutes. Rinse with warm water.

Main ingredient: peppermint

Peppermint reduces sebum production without drying out the skin. It also balances the skin's pH levels to prevent acne, pimples, and blackheads.

Creamy Thyme Face Mask

Ingredients: 1 tablespoon sour cream, 1 tablespoon fresh thyme leaves, 1 teaspoon unfiltered raw honey, ½ teaspoon lemon juice

Directions: Put all the ingredients in a blender or food processor. Process until the thyme leaves is shredded in tiny pieces. Apply the mask to a clean face and leave on for 10-15 minutes. Rinse well with warm water.

Main ingredient: thyme

When it comes to healing acne, thyme's properties greatly rival the benzoyl peroxide. It cleanses the skin, removes deep-seated dirt, and reduces any swelling. Importantly, it doesn't have any side effects compared to other pimple-fight chemical product.

Veggie Facial Mask

Ingredients: 1 teaspoon parsley, 1 teaspoon cucumber (unpeeled), and 1 teaspoon yogurt

Directions: Place all the ingredients in a blender. Process until creamy. Massage on clean skin and leave on for 15 minutes. Rinse with lukewarm water.

Main ingredient: cucumber

Cucumber naturally reduces appearance of dark eye circles and puffy eyes. It also soothes the skin, improves the skin's complexion, fades facial scars, and minimizes pore size.

Tomato Oatmeal Mask

Ingredients: 1 teaspoon rolled oats, 1 teaspoon lemon juice, and 1 ripe tomato

Directions: Place all the ingredients in a blender. Process until a fine mush is achieved. Apply on clean skin and leave on for 30 minutes. Wipe off with a damp washcloth before rinsing with cold water.

Main ingredient: tomato

Tomatoes delay skin aging and appearance of wrinkles. Full of vitamin C, it gets rid of blackheads, dries out acne, and heal acne-related wounds and infections.

Breakout Busting Mask

Ingredients: 3 drops fresh lemon juice, 1 teaspoon raw honey, and 1 teaspoon ground cloves

Directions: Mix all the ingredients in a small bowl. Apply on the face and leave to dry. Rinse with lukewarm water.

Main ingredient: ground clove

Ground clove contains anti-inflammatory properties that reduce acne swelling. It also evens out complexion and exfoliates the skin to bring out a wonderful glow.

Bay Leaf Clay Mask

Ingredients: 5 dried bay leaves, 4 tablespoons French green clay, and 1 cup distilled water

Directions: Boil the water and put in the bay leaves. Let steep for 10 minutes and let cool Discard the leaves and add in the clay. Once a paste is formed, apply on the face and allow to dry. Rinse with warm water.

Main ingredient: bay leaves

Bay leaves liven up tired and stressed skin. It reduces appearances of fine line and acne outbreaks. Its healing properties heal insect bites and stings and bacterial infections.

Chapter 6: Facial Mask for Dry and Sensitive Skin

For Dry Skin

Lemon Egg Mask

Ingredients: 1 egg yolk, 1 teaspoon turmeric powder, and 1 teaspoons olive oil

Directions: Whisk the egg yolk and add in the turmeric. Add the olive oil slowly. Mix well. Apply the mask on face and neck. Leave on the face until dry. Wipe off with a damp, warm washcloth. Rinse with cold water.

Main ingredient: egg yolk

Egg yolks contain zinc, vitamin A, vitamin B2, and vitamin B3 that help reduce swelling, heal minute cracks and wounds, and soften and moisturize skin. Constant application of this facial mask also brightens the skin and evens skin tone.

Flour Mayo Mask

Ingredients: 4 teaspoons gram flour, 2 teaspoons wheat flour, 1 tablespoon mayonnaise and 4 tablespoons honey

Directions: Place all in the ingredients in the blender. Process until thick. Apply on the face and leave on for 20 minutes before rinsing with cool water.

Main ingredient: mayonnaise

Mayonnaise contains eggs, soybean oil, and vinegar which are quite beneficial for the skin. The eggs and soybean oil effectively moisturizes skin and while the vinegar encourages skin cell regeneration to make skin brighter.

Strawberry and Papaya Mask

Ingredients: 1 peach (cooked), 2 fresh strawberries (large), ½ very ripe papaya, 1 tablespoon oatmeal, and 1 teaspoon honey (organic)

Directions: Place all the fruits in a bowl. Mash and mix together. Stir in the oatmeal and until thick paste is formed. Apply on the face and leave on for 15 minutes. Rinse with warm water.

Main ingredients: strawberry and papaya

Strawberries contain vitamin C, natural exfoliants, and antioxidants which tighten pores, remove impurities, soften skin. It also lightens age spots and freckles. Papaya keeps the skin hydrated and supple because it doesn't contain any sodium. It also slows down skin aging.

Fennel Seed Mask

Ingredients: 1 tablespoon fennel seeds, 1 tablespoon honey, and 1 tablespoon oatmeal

Directions: Steep the fennel seeds in ½ cup of boiling water for 10 minutes. Strain the liquid and let cool. Grind the oatmeal using a food processor. Add the ground oatmeal to the fennel tea. Mix in the honey. Apply on the face and rinse after 20 minutes with tepid and cold water.

Main ingredient: Fennel seed

Fennel effectively regulates the skin's moisture level to make the skin supple and moisturized. It also stimulates the blood circulation which make the skin toned, elastic, and smooth.

Aloe Vera Mask

Ingredients: 1 teaspoon aloe vera juice, ½ teaspoon jojoba oil, 2 tablespoons of green clay, 1 drop lavender oil, and 1 drop bergamot oil

Directions: Combine all the ingredients and stir well. Add a few drops of water to make a paste. Apply on the face and leave on for 15 minutes. Rinse off with warm water.

Main ingredients: aloe vera juice

Aloe vera moisturizes the skin without making the skin overly greasy. It also reduces skin inflammation, reduces fine lines, and minimizes facial scarring.

For Sensitive Skin

Avocado Yogurt Mask

Ingredients: ½ cup yogurt (plain, not non-fat), ¼ cup honey, and 1 very ripe avocado

Directions: Slice the avocado open. Remove the seed and remove the flesh of the avocado. Place the avocado meat in the bowl and mash it in chunks. Mix in the yogurt and honey. Stir well. Apply the mask on a clean face and leave for 30 minutes. Rinse off with warm water.

Main ingredient: avocado and yogurt

The avocado fruit is rich in vitamin A, vitamin D, and vitamin E. All these vitamins help keep the skin healthy, young, and moisturized. The yogurt contains various enzymes, zinc and protein that helps cleanse and soften skin.

Rose Clay Mask

Ingredients: 1 tablespoon rose clay, 1 drop rose oil, 2 teaspoons avocado oil, 1 drop Roman chamomile oil

Directions: Combine all the ingredients in a bowl. Add a few drops of water to create a paste. Apply on clean face and let dry. Rinse off with warm water and, then cold water.

Main ingredient: rose clay

A mild kaolin clay, rose clay gently cleanses and exfoliates the skin by removing dead skin cells and opening clogged pores. It also improves the blood circulation on the face and gives it a rosy, pink glow.

Cornmeal Chamomile Mask

Ingredients: 1 tablespoon freshly brewed chamomile tea, and 1 teaspoon milk powder, and 1 teaspoon cornmeal

Directions: Pour the chamomile tea in a bowl and slowly add in the milk powder. Stir well before adding the cornmeal. Once a paste is formed, apply on the skin and leave on for 10 minutes. Rinse with warm water.

Main ingredient: chamomile tea

Chamomile tea contains antioxidants that prevent acne and future breakouts. It also provides a natural, pinkish glow.

Conclusion

Thank you again for purchasing this book!

I hope this book was able to help you make easy and effective body scrubs and facial masks.

The next step is to experiment further with various natural ingredients. Just simply enjoy the scrubs' scent and the relaxing feel that they offer whenever you use them.

Finally, if you enjoyed this book, please take the time to share your thoughts and post a review on Amazon. We do our best to reach out to readers and provide the best value we can. Your positive review will help us achieve that. It'd be greatly appreciated!

Thank you and good luck!

Check Out My Other Books

Below you'll find some of my other popular books that are popular on Amazon and Kindle as well. Simply click on the links below to check them out. Alternatively, you can visit my author page on Amazon to see other work done by me.

Coconut Oil for Easy Weight Loss: A Step by Step Guide for Using Virgin Coconut Oil for Quick and Easy Weight Loss

http://www.amazon.com/Coconut-Oil-Easy-Weight-Loss-ebook/dp/B00JG8H8DE

Superfoods that Kickstart Your Weight Loss Learn How to Use 30 Superfoods to Boost Weight Loss, Immunity and to Live a Healthier Lifestyle

http://www.amazon.com/Superfoods-that-Kickstart-Your-Weight-ebook/dp/B00JNAPM9M

Carrier Oils for Beginners: Discover the Characteristics and Beauty and Health Benefits of Carrier Oils For mixing Aromatherapy Essential Oils

http://www.amazon.com/Carrier-Oils-Beginners-Characteristics-Aromatherapy-ebook/dp/B00K88GI2S

Natural Homemade Cleaning Recipes For Beginners: Essential Oil Recipes For Household Cleaning, Laundry & Toxic Free Living

http://www.amazon.com/Natural-Homemade-Cleaning-Recipes-Beginners-ebook/dp/B00K87UBQI

The Best Secrets of Natural Remedies: The Ultimate Guide to Natural Remedies to Prevent and Cure Illnesses, Cold and Flu for Your Family

http://www.amazon.com/Best-Secrets-Natural-Remedies-Illnesses-ebook/dp/B00JNDCOCM

The Hypothyroidism Handbook:An Everyday Guide to Natural Solutions of living with Hypothyroidism including increased energy, lasting weight loss, and general well-being

http://www.amazon.com/Hypothyroidism-Handbook-Solutions-including-increased-ebook/dp/B00JNIGIV0

The Hyperthyroidism Handbook: An Everyday Guide to Natural Solutions of Living with Hyperthyroidism including Weight Gain, Increased Energy and General Well-being

http://www.amazon.com/Hyperthyroidism-Handbook-Solutions-including-Hypothyroidism-ebook/dp/B00JOHU5SM

Essential Oils & Weight Loss for Beginners: Ultimate Guide to Losing Weight, Increasing Energy, Balancing Metabolism & Appetite Using Essential Oils & Aromatherapy

http://www.amazon.com/Essential-Oils-Weight-Loss-Beginners-ebook/dp/B00JOFOWP6

Top Essential Oil Recipes: A Recipe Guide Of Natural, Non-Toxic Aromatherapy & Essential Oils for Healing Common Ailments, Beauty, Stress & Anxiety

http://www.amazon.com/Top-Essential-Oil-Recipes-Aromatherapy-ebook/dp/B00JY434E2

Soap Making For Beginners: A Guide to Making Natural Homemade Soaps from Scratch, Includes Recipes and Step by Step Processes for Making Soaps

http://www.amazon.com/Soap-Making-Beginners-Homemade-Processes-ebook/dp/B00JYKH75I

Body Butters For Beginners: Proven Secrets To Making All Natural Body Butters For Rejuvenating And Hydrating Your Skin

http://www.amazon.com/Body-Butters-Beginners-Rejuvenating-Hydrating-ebook/dp/B00K6LVV6A

Apple Cider Vinegar For Beginners: Proven Secrets Using Apple Cider Vinegar For Health, Weight Loss, and Skin Care

http://www.amazon.com/Apple-Cider-Vinegar-Beginners-Aromatherapy-ebook/dp/B00K6YY6HI

Homemade Body Scrubs & Masks For Beginners: 50 Proven All Natural, Easy Recipes For Body & Facial Masks To Exfoliate Nourish, & Care For Your Skin

http://www.amazon.com/Homemade-Body-Scrubs-Masks-Beginners-ebook/dp/B00K79D4SY

Essential Oils Box Set #1: Essential Oils & Weight Loss For Beginners (Ultimate Guide to Losing Weight, Increasing Energy, Balancing Metabolism & Appetite Using Essential Oils & Aromatherapy) + Top Essential Oil Recipes (A Recipe Guide of Natural, Non-Toxic Aromatherapy & Essential Oils for Healing Common Ailments, Beauty, Stress & Anxiety)

http://www.amazon.com/ESSENTIAL-OILS-BOX-SET-Aromatherapy-ebook/dp/B00K7Q8HRK

Essential Oils Box Set #2: Essential Oils & Weight Loss For Beginners (Ultimate Guide to Losing Weight, Increasing Energy, Balancing Metabolism & Appetite Using Essential Oils & Aromatherapy) + Top Essential Oil Recipes (A Recipe Guide of Natural, Non-Toxic Aromatherapy & Essential Oils for Healing Common Ailments, Beauty, Stress & Anxiety)

http://www.amazon.com/ESSENTIAL-OILS-BOX-SET-Aromatherapy-ebook/dp/B00K7Q8HRK

Box Set#3: Coconut Oil for Easy Weight Loss(A Step by Step Guide for Using Virgin Coconut Oil for Quick and Easy Weight Loss) + Apple Cider Vinegar(Proven Secrets Using Apple Cider Vinegar for Health, Weight Loss, and Skin Care)

http://www.amazon.com/Box-Set-Beginners-Aromatherapy-Essential-ebook/dp/B00K9TEGUW

Box Set #4: Body butters For Beginners(Proven Secrets To Making All Natural Body Butters For Rejuvenating And Hydrating Your Skin) & Top Essential Oil Recipes: A Recipe Guide Of Natural, Non-Toxic Aromatherapy & Essential Oils for Healing Common Ailments, Beauty, Stress & Anxiety http://www.amazon.com/Box-Set-Butters-Beginners-Essential-ebook/dp/B00KA02F4Y

Box Set #5: Soap Making For Beginners(A Guide to Making Natural Homemade Soaps from Scratch, Includes Recipes and Step by Step Processes for Making Soaps) + Homemade Body Scrubs & Masks For Beginners(50 Proven All Natural, Easy Recipes For Body Scrub & Facial Masks To Efoliate, Nourish, & Care For Your Skin)

http://www.amazon.com/Box-Set-Beginners-Homemade-Recipes-ebook/dp/B00K9U3I2I

Box Set #6: Body Butters for Beginners (Proven Secrets To Making All Natural Body Butters For Rejuvenating And Hydrating Your Skin) +Homemade Body Scrubs & Masks For Beginners(50 Proven All Natural, Easy Recipes For Body Scrub & Facial Masks To Exfoliate, Nourish, & Care For Your Skin)

http://www.amazon.com/Box-Set-Beginners-Exfoliating-Moisturizing-ebook/dp/B00K9U3Y4O

Box Set #7: TOP ESSENTIAL OILS(A Recipe Guide Of Natural, Non-Toxic Aromatherapy & Essential Oils For Healing, Common Ailments, Beauty, Stress & Anxiety) & THE BEST SECRETS OF NATURAL REMEDIES(The Ultimate Guide to Natural Remedies to Prevent and Cure Illnesses, Cold and Flu for Your Family)

http://www.amazon.com/BOX-SET-Essential-Recipes-Remedies-ebook/dp/B00K9WPMQG

Box Set #8: NATURAL HOMEMADE CLEANING RECIPES FOR BEGINNERS (Essential Oil Recipes for Household Cleaning, Laundry & Toxic Free Living) + TOP ESSENTIAL OILS(A Recipe Guide Of Natural, Non-Toxic Aromatherapy & Essential Oils For Healing, Common Ailments, Beauty, Stress & Anxiety)

http://www.amazon.com/BOX-SET-Beginners-Essential-Aromatherapy-ebook/dp/B00KAMNGBS

Box Set #9: Essential Oils & Weight Loss for Beginners (Ultimate Guide to Losing Weight, Increasing Energy, Balancing Metabolism & Appetite Using Essential Oils & Aromatherapy) + Carrier Oils for Beginners (Discover the Characteristics and Beauty and Health Benefits of Carrier Oils for Mixing Aromatherapy Essential Oils)

http://www.amazon.com/BOX-SET-Essential-Beginners-Aromatherapy-ebook/dp/B00KAODL6Q

BOX SET #10: THE HYPERTHYROIDISM HANDBOOK (An Everyday Guide to Natural Solutions of Living with Hyperthyroidism including Weight Gain, Increased Energy and General Well-being) + THE HYPOTHYROIDISM HANDBOOK (Everyday Guide to Natural Solutions of Living With Hypothyroidism Including Increased Energy, Lasting Weight Loss, and General Well-Being)

http://www.amazon.com/BOX-SET-10-Hyperthyroidism-Hypothyroidism-ebook/dp/B00KAKMSBY

BOX SET #11: CARRIER OILS FOR BEGINNERS (Discover the Characteristics and Beauty and Health Benefits of Carrier Oils for Mixing Aromatherapy Essential Oils) + Essential Oils & Aromatherapy for Beginners (Secrets to Beauty, Health and Weight Loss Using Proven Essential Oil and Aromatherapy Recipes

http://www.amazon.com/BOX-SET-Beginners-Essential-Aromatherapy-ebook/dp/B00KAONEQ8

BOX SET 12: ESSENTIAL OILS & WEIGHT LOSS FOR BEGINNERS: (Ultimate Guide to Losing Weight, Increasing Energy, Balancing Metabolism & Appetite Using Essential Oils & Aromatherapy) + TOP ESSENTIAL OIL RECIPES (A Recipe Guide of Natural, Non-Toxic Aromatherapy & Essential Oils for Healing Common Ailments, Beauty, Stress & Anxiety) + CARRIER OILS FOR BEGINNERS (Discover the Characteristics & Beauty & Health Benefits of Carrier Oils for Mixing Aromatherapy Essential Oils) + ESSENTIAL OILS & AROMATHERAPY FOR BEGINNERS (Secrets to Beauty & weight Loss Using Proven Essential Oil & Aromatherapy Recipes) + NATURAL HOMEMADE CLEANING RECIPES FOR BEGINNERS (Essential Oil Recipes for Household Cleaning, Laundry & Toxic Free Living)

http://www.amazon.com/BOX-SET-12-Essential-Aromatherapy-ebook/dp/B00KCBCHE4

BOX SET #13: SUPERFOODS THAT KICKSTART YOUR WEIGHT LOSS (Learn How to Use 30 Superfoods to Boost Weight Loss, Immunity and to Live a Healthier Lifestyle) + ESSENTIAL OILS & AROMATHERAPY FOR BEGINNERS (Secrets to Beauty, Health and Weight Loss Using Proven Essential Oil and Aromatherapy Recipes) + BODY BUTTERS FOR BEGINNERS (Proven Secrets To Making All Natural Body

Butters For Rejuvenating And Hydrating Your Skin) + SOAP MAKING FOR BEGINNERS (A Guide to Making Natural Homemade Soaps from Scratch, Includes Recipes and Step by Step Processes for Making Soaps) + HOMEMADE BODY SCRUBS FOR BEGINNERS (50 Proven All Natural, Easy Recipes For Body Scrub & Facial Masks To Exfoliate, Nourish, & Care For Your Skin)

http://www.amazon.com/BOX-SET-Superfoods-Kickstart-Aromatherapy-ebook/dp/B00KC8G6DK/

BOX SET 14: Essential Oils & Weight Loss for Beginners (Ultimate Guide to Losing Weight, Increasing Energy, Balancing Metabolism & Appetite Using Essential Oils & Aromatherapy) + Apple Cider Vinegar for Beginners (Proven Secrets Using Apple Cider Vinegar for Health, Weight Loss, and Skin Care) + Body Butters For Beginners (Proven Secrets To Making All Natural Body Butters For Rejuvenating And Hydrating Your Skin)
+ Homemade Body Scrubs & Masks for Beginners (50 Proven All Natural, Easy Recipes for Body Scrub & Facial Masks to Exfoliate, Nourish, & Care for Your Skin) + Coconut Oil for Easy Weight Loss (A Step by Step Guide for Using Virgin Coconut Oil for Quick and Easy Weight Loss)

http://www.amazon.com/BOX-SET-Essential-Beginners-Aromatherapy-ebook/dp/B00KEDO68U

If the links do not work, for whatever reason, you can simply search for these titles on the Amazon website to find them.

www.ingramcontent.com/pod-product-compliance
Lightning Source LLC
Chambersburg PA
CBHW060312290526
45789CB00001B/491